Ethical and Aesthetic Explorations of Systemic Practice

In *Ethical and Aesthetic Explorations of Systemic Practice*, the four co-authors come together to rhizomatically consider how systemic theories can be reinvigorated in the present day.

This fascinating book uses the ideas and work of renowned anthropologist Gregory Bateson as a springboard from which to examine the fundamental tenets of systemic theory and practice, as well as looking to the work of Deleuze, Guattari, Maturana, Varela and von Foerster. Including contributions from a range of renowned therapists, each chapter examines the guiding principles from a critical perspective, asking questions around the ontology of the therapeutic encounter and the technique of therapy itself.

This revivifying volume will be of interest to systemic professionals, and those looking at how the systemic community can continue to grow and evolve.

Pietro Barbetta is a psychotherapist, Director of the Milan Center of Family Therapy and Professor of Psychodynamic Theories at Bergamo University, Italy. He also works as an ethno-clinical therapist with asylum seekers and refugees, and has authored works in English, Italian, Spanish and French.

Maria Esther Cavagnis is the Director of Studies, Clinical Research Team Coordinator and Senior Tutor in the therapist training program at the Family Therapy Foundation in Buenos Aires, Argentina. She is a visiting lecturer at several universities in Argentina and Latin America and has worked in private practice since 1982.

Inga-Britt Krause is a social anthropologist, Consultant Systemic Psychotherapist and Lead of the Professional Doctorate in Systemic Psychotherapy at The Tavistock & Portman NHS Foundation Trust, UK. She is an international systemic psychotherapy teacher, trainer and supervisor, Visiting Professor in Social Anthropology at the University of Oslo, and consultant to several contemporary anthropological research projects.

Umberta Telfener is a teacher at the Milan School of Family Therapy, Italy and is Chair of the European Family Therapy Association Training Institutes Chamber (EFTA-TIC). Formerly Adjunct Professor at the Health Psychology Postgraduate School of the University of Rome La Sapienza, she has supervised public mental health structures and worked in private practice since 1982. She has authored works in both English and Italian.

The Systemic Thinking and Practice Series

Series Editors
Charlotte Burck and Gwyn Daniel

This influential series was co-founded in 1989 by series editors David Campbell and Ros Draper to promote innovative applications of systemic theory to psychotherapy, teaching, supervision and organisational consultation. In 2011, Charlotte Burck and Gwyn Daniel became series editors and aim to present new theoretical developments and pioneering practice, to make links with other theoretical approaches, and to promote the relevance of systemic theory to contemporary social and psychological questions.

Recent titles in the series include:

Creativity in Times of Constraint: A Practitioner's Companion in Mental Health and Social Care
Jim Wilson

Staying Attached: Fathers and Children in Troubled Times
Gill Gorell Barnes

The Heart of the Matter: Music and Art in Family Therapy
Hilary Palmer

Family Dramas: Intimacy, Power and Systems in Shakespeare's Tragedies
Gwyn Daniel

The Times of Time: A Perspective on Time in Systemic Therapy and Consultation
Luigi Boscolo and Paolo Bertrando

Ethical and Aesthetic Explorations of Systemic Practice: New Critical Reflections
Pietro Barbetta, Maria Esther Cavagnis, Inga-Britt Krause and Umberta Telfener

Ethical and Aesthetic Explorations of Systemic Practice

New Critical Reflections

Pietro Barbetta, Maria Esther Cavagnis, Inga-Britt Krause and Umberta Telfener

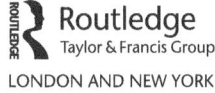
Routledge
Taylor & Francis Group

LONDON AND NEW YORK

Cover image: "Returning Together" (detail) by David Hobson

First published 2022
by Routledge
4 Park Square, Milton Park, Abingdon, Oxon OX14 4RN

and by Routledge
605 Third Avenue, New York, NY 10158

Routledge is an imprint of the Taylor & Francis Group, an informa business

British Library Cataloguing-in-Publication Data
A catalogue record for this book is available from the British Library

Library of Congress Cataloging-in-Publication Data
A catalog record has been requested for this book

ISBN: 978-1-138-34619-2 (hbk)
ISBN: 978-1-138-34621-5 (pbk)
ISBN: 978-0-429-43741-0 (ebk)

DOI: 10.4324/9780429437410

Typeset in Times New Roman
by Taylor & Francis Books

Contents

Series Editors' Foreword
Charlotte Burck and Gwyn Daniel

It is a particular pleasure to include in our series a book which does so much to push the conceptual frontiers within our field. This volume is a tour de force, the result of intellectual journeys at many diverse levels and in many disciplines as well as of enriching conversations and collaborations between the four authors. They aim to rekindle some of the pioneering and creative spirit of earlier developments in systemic therapy and they do this by staking out a position of observing and questioning – as if from outside – the ortho-doxies that have evolved over the decades. In doing so they re-animate the ideas of curiosity, ethics and aesthetics. The book provides valuable and innovative commentaries on the radical work of Deleuze and Guattari, draws upon the field of social anthropology and provides other perspectives from philosophy, film and drama. The authors are rigorous in their exploration of language and discourse in the systemic field, both in critiquing the ways in which language constrains and in their adaptation of linguistic forms from philosophy and other fields, some of which will be as new to the reader as they were to the series editors.

A major part of the book involves a re-examination of the work of Gregory Bateson and a recovery of his pioneering anthropological work. The rigorous ongoing questioning of ethical positions and their theoretical underpinnings and, above all, the ability to link such enquiries to dilemmas within clinical practice is one of the strengths of the book and an invaluable aid to therapists in reflecting on their work within different contexts. This book discusses theory and clinical examples in a way that connects ethics and aesthetics and which is acutely aware of the dynamics of power and the possibilities for lib-eratory practice. Another great strength of this book is that it includes a focus on work with both adults and children and across cultures and clinical contexts.

The authors describe developing their thinking together as a cross-cultural collective which continues to be distinguished by and in their differences, expecting, in their words, "gaps and distances to be travelled such as has been the case in the writing of this book". The reader hopefully will have the experience too of joining a conversation in which they will experience provocations to expand their frameworks of thinking.

In keeping with the processes enacted so creatively between the authors, some of the central conceptualizations coalesce around ideas such as mapping, cartography, trajectories, lines of flight and processes of becoming, and thus speak so well to our times when migration in all its various forms is one of the key socio/political/psychological experiences. These ideas challenge us in our therapeutic activity and will hopefully invite readers to think anew and feel reinvigorated.

We are delighted and privileged to include this volume in our series.

Charlotte Burck
Gwyn Daniel
December 2021

Chapter 1

Introduction

Why Ethic and Aesthetic in Systemic Practices

Pietro Barbetta, Maria Esther Cavagnis,
Inga Britt Krause and Umberta Telfener

How to Introduce a Book that Aims to Critically Explore the World of Systemic Practice?

The clinic is a world in itself, populated by many styles, each with their own recognizable tunes. Practice – clinical practice – is a word that is familiar to clinicians; perhaps too familiar to support an engagement with it in a curious way. Not the curiosity that is now paradoxically institutionalized in the training of systemic therapists but the curiosity that informed Bateson (1979) and the impetus of the word "systemic" as an epistemic alternative to mainstream ideas in the social sciences. This book wants to connect with that spirit, with the search of different territories for a systemic practice. Throughout the last 45 years, systemic practices have been entangled within different kinds of frames, strategic, structural, social constructionist, narrative, etc. Nonetheless, in our view, all the frames we mentioned have a kind of transcendental premise: the strategic model hides the premise that the therapist should win the (psychotic) game; the structural model seems to recommend the reverence to generational hierarchies; social constructionism has the naïve idea of "collaborative" practice as linguistic practice, taking for granted that "collaboration" is a "good practice"; narrative model frames the person within a character of the narrative, like in a text. War, hierarchy, collaboration and textuality are the ways in which the systemic models have framed the systemic practice.

In this book we foster an out-of-frame approach, based on the difference between epistemology and ontology. An ongoing reflecting search for the multiple senses of reality.

Such a search might require us, as it did with Bateson (1979), to carefully re-engage with the order of the things, as Foucault (2001) would say, so as to look at its interstices in search of differences. Rather than going up into new interpretative worlds, we are interested in staying in the immanent plane where theory and practice meet and engage in a stochastic process, where the final outcome is not known (Bateson, 1979). Such an exploration needs not only to clarify – shed light – but also has to move/transform the position from

DOI: 10.4324/9780429437410-1

which we started the exploration. Such a *search with a difference* requires us to start somewhere, not because origins are important per se but because such a gesture helps us recognize the material dimension of the exploration. As we stated, this is not a book aiming to identify abstract possibilities but to engage with material conditions in search of transformation, going back to the origins and, through this (re)turn, reinventing them. In this case, the materiality we want to explore is that of clinical practice, in particular, the insights that Bateson and subsequent systemic thinkers have proposed for the work in the clinic. At the same time there are authors not usually thought of as systemic thinkers, but whose work can contribute to this "reading back" and who sometimes seem to be nearer to Bateson than some contemporary systemic psychotherapists. We are thinking here of writers such as Gilles Deleuze and Felix Guattari (1987), Michel Foucault (2001) and some social anthropologists who followed their paths. In this introductory chapter we offer the premise of the following book. Coherence is not necessarily what we are looking for; to the contrary we had a very long period of conversation about styles and approaches, with the aim, as in the title, to give the reader an ethic and aesthetic approach to systemic *practice*.

Practicare

Such an exploration needs to start somewhere and we feel that it is useful to begin with the word *practice*. *Practice* is a polysemic word with a proliferation of meanings, or, to be more precise, *practice* is a word which produces a differentiation between meaning and sense, concept and expression, ethic and aesthetic. As a concept, *practice* has to do with ethics; as an expression, it deals with living experience, from the Greek word *aisthesis*, meaning sensorial, perceptual and corporeal experience. There are multiple facets of practice: dominant and dissident ones. From Greek, *praktiké* is considered the part of philosophy concerning the action – versus *gnostiké*, what concerns knowledge. During the Enlightenment and in Romantic philosophy, practice had to do with ethics and aesthetics; starting from Marx, in social philosophy the word "praxis" became the way of going out from interpretation and focusing on transformation (Marx and Engels, 1998). A similar idea, in genealogic sense, comes from Nietzsche – how to do philosophy with the hammer (Nietzsche, 2005) – while in modern phenomenology, there is a distinction between essence and existence (Satre, 1943) where what one theorizes as essence is far from what one does in existence.

Within the aesthetics of complexity, the concept of "enaction" (Varela et al., 2017) indicates a different form of knowledge, not categorial or abstract, like the one we are used to learning within school and academia. It is rather an intuition, which appears in conjunction with an event. Something that does not appear within the realm of necessity, nor within the realm of possibility (or probability). It rather is a third kind of knowledge, which appears in the dominion of contingency: the frog eats flies, at the same time frogs do not simply eat flies, they eat this particular fly that is flying, on the visual panorama of the frog. Cognition is not awareness, it is rather acquaintance, something corporeal, which belongs to the body. This kind of knowledge makes series proliferate; enaction seems to be the condition for producing lines of flight (hospitality, art, literature, music are all practices), or, vice versa, for oppression (restraint, torture, death penalty, abuses are also practices).

It is clear that, in practice, ethics matter. What does systemic practice mean, not only in therapy, but also in research, teaching, training and other different fields of experience? In what way can the authors define what it means, for example, to use the term "practitioner"? The authors of this book have enough experience in systemic therapy. They have been involved as subjects and practitioners in cultural dissonance, multi-perspective therapeutic and political experiences. We are particularly interested in those aspects of critical systemic work that – despite being central to the work – have been neglected, if not forgotten, by mainstream approaches. This is why we have gathered together these few voices who are all inspired to try to think about what might or can be different. In line with the second engagement with Bateson by the therapists at the Milan Group from the 1980s on (Boscolo et al., 1987), this book intends to offer a reading that engages with practice as an ethical and aesthetical activity rather than transcendental "linguistic games", or "social constructions". *Practice* has been with us for a long time. According to etymological dictionaries, it emerged in the English vocabulary early in the fifteenth century from variations of the Old French *pratiser* and Medieval Latin *practicare*. It is hard to know what was first, whether it was first a noun followed by its use as a verb and an adjective or whether these permutations were of a different order. What we can say is that by 1600, the word was used in all these Porfirian registers to refer to the application and the effectuation of ideas.

In this focus on the etymology of the word, we can already see the order of the discourse (Foucault, 1971a) that is established surrounding the word *practice* and its derivatives. In line with the often uncritically assumed linguistic structure of our knowledge – the (in)famous image of the tree of knowledge – the emerging relationship between ourselves and the world of which we are making sense needs not just a theory but also a practice and, in such necessity, our thoughts are pushed into action. Although too early in the exploration, we are already dissatisfied with what we see as a problematic and unexamined relationship with etymology and with the term *practice*. We feel there is something missing if we approach considerations on practice solely through definitions in themselves, even when we do so taking into account historical descriptions of their origins. We do not want to dismiss the value of these activities. That is, we do feel it is important to both define something, to punctuate the flow of everyday life and provide it with a certain shape, as well as to look at its etymology, that is to look at the variations and movements that such punctuation has had through time. Even when we focus on the case of the verb *practice* – a verb being that part of discourse which designates actions thus conveying an implicit space for movement and possibility – there is an absence in the definition for the space that always presents itself in the contingent and the unexpected. What we are trying to grasp in our exploration is not a new territory that has been established in the therapeutic world with the creation of a new name – family therapy – but the process of exploring and expanding the definitions that were at the base of such emergence. We are – as we explained earlier – stubbornly sticking to the surface of the systemic gesture, to the encounter with what is contingent and accidental.

Poiesis

It is in this sense and through these transformations that *practice*, from a systemic perspective, needs a new conceptualization as a de-generate and uncanny word. *Systemic practice* then not only deals with a certain position and place in the discourse – *practice* – but also has to deal with the actuality of what is "contingent", with an openness to, a facing at, the un-usual. It is in fact this latter part, this aspect of practice that faces us with something that one cannot use in the usual way – the interstices of the definition of practice – that we feel is central to what is systemic.

Practice becomes an autopoietic concept in that it needs to constantly produce its own definition in front of what is presented in its space. Practice in the clinic is a fundamentally critical and creative exercise that needs to engage, not with what is familiar and predictable, but with the singularity present in the contingency of the event that is presented to the clinic. Such an engagement is revolutionary in the sense used by Deleuze and Foucault because it is, simultaneously, an engagement with the current discourse and its disruption. In such a gesture, systemic practice pursues supporting the becoming of the event; of the possibilities of life imbued in the presentation of a client and his/her/their moment of life in the clinic. Systemic practice then is not only uncanny but also unhinging. Following these considerations, there are, in the contemporary context, a number of significant questions that demand to be asked.

Scientia

Is systemic practice scientific? If it is so, what kind of science is it? Is it reproducible or reliable? Or is it a kind of idiosyncratic approach, which deals with people who have particular kinds of esoteric experiences? Is it a kind of art? Is it something else? From a systemic perspective, sciences continually attempt to falsify their own hypotheses. As in the Milan Approach, science is something in which one of the ethical imperatives is "never fall in love with your own hypotheses" (Cecchin, 1987) The science of the systemic practice is composed by dissident words: accountability vs reliability, difference in repetition vs mere repetition of the same practice (as in bureaucracy), hypotheses coming from the singular history vs standard diagnostic verifiability. It is in this sense that a re-engagement with systemic practice and science can be best done through an engagement with the ideas of Foucault, Deleuze and others who are rarely listed in current professional definitions. Foucault's active renaming of his Chair at the College de France as History of Systems of Thought (Foucault, 1971a) is an important gesture in this sense. In order to understand the limits of the current discourse of scientific blind-ness that takes place in current clinical practice, it is important to learn from literature, anthropology, philosophy, and arts, as well as from studying the history of systems of care and cure from the ancient theory of moods (from Hippocrates to late Renaissance), to the modern diagnosis (from Thomas Wills to the DSM-5).

In this sense, for instance, the way in which alchemists such as Paracelsus used the Magic Square to cure melancholia, or the African Marabou use rituals to heal grievances of the body and the mind, have to be observed and studied. Such a knowledge is crucial to identify the interstices of the prevalence of evidence-based practice dominant in the current pharmacy-psychiatric environment, evidence that uncritically relies on "universal diagnosis" and that insidiously screens people through a grid-inventory, positioning them effectively into subjects, *subjugated* and *docile* bodies within the same cage. Instead Deleuze invites us to disrupt the monolithic language of science by questioning the presence of different types of sciences, one serving the purpose of the State and one that is minor and nomadic. Such a science is not a science of grids and of docile bodies but a "science of becoming" (Cecchin et al., 2005; von Foerster, 1995)

Nomadic Science

It is not by chance that the most important point of reference for systemic practice is Gregory Bateson. He was an anthropologist (Bateson, 1958),[1] neither a psychiatrist nor a psychologist. This means that his gaze on therapy was from the outside. Regarding therapy, Bateson's gaze is like "a thought from outside", to mention the title of a book written by Foucault, dedicated to Maurice Blanchot (1987). It is as if someone comes and observes something from a different perspective, from another field, which never faced what she/he is going to observe right now. This was the role of Bateson at the Paolo Alto Veteran Hospital. The psychiatric staff invited Bateson to take up such a role. Bateson had always been a nomadic person, a kind of *flaneur* among different disciplines; this is probably the reason why Gilles Deleuze claimed that he was a genius (Deleuze, 2014). Deleuze and Guattari (1987) used the word "nomadic" to define a particular kind of way of living. *Homo Sapiens/ Demens* is a nomadic animal by definition, it settles down here and there for a short period of time pretending to be the landlord of the territory it occupies as settler. Migration has always been the most important activity of such an animal from the origins. Starting from Bateson, systemic practice moved in-between different territories of knowledge and action: biology, neurology, mathematics, sociology, ethology, psychotherapy and arts. During a conference Bateson told the students that, although at university they are taught to separate anthropology from sociology, and both from psychology, and all these fields from literature and arts, the reality is a connection between all these subjects. But systemic is much more than just a multidisciplinary approach; it is also epistemology and ontology, a way of seeing and engaging with the world.

This book aims to identify new directions in systemic practice. It aims to engage with the systemic gesture as it has emerged out of the work of some of the critical thinkers – like Bateson, Foucault and Deleuze – who share an immanent view of life in ways that honor current sensitivities in terms of critical thinking. Over many years there has been a group of Bateson followers and associates who developed his way of thinking, and applied it to different fields: Humberto Maturana, Francisco Varela, Heinz von Foerster, to mention only a few. They created key concepts like "autopoiesis", "enaction", "perturbation", "order from noise", "non-trivial machines", and those concepts have had the role of supplementing Gregory Bateson's thought in a way that made a revolution in cybernetics. Those thinkers called this new way of practicing "second-order cybernetics". Other sources of our inspiration, particularly coming from European philosophy, are: Ronald Laing (1961) and others who were in touch with Bateson for brief periods, inspired by him; those who, even not knowing him personally, used his thoughts in different ways and perspectives; or those who have done similar work, apparently in different ways, but actually converging with the systemic field.

Clinics

The classical clinical theory in psychotherapy has been widely reduced to a simple and unique story: the subject is the person who is no longer adaptable within the family, and is dysfunctional in society. He/she is not integrated into the usual circumstances of life, no longer prompted to obtain new goals, losing job and credibility in society. Psychotherapy (family therapy, individual therapy, psychoanalysis) became the practices of working with the latent structure of the Ego for providing new "energy" in order to make the Ego stronger, more aware, adaptable, goal oriented and integrated into the modern society. It is a matter of reinforcing the defensive mechanisms of the Ego, or dismantling them when dysfunctional – providing other, more functional, mechanisms. The goal of the treatment was repairing subjects from homosexuality, hyper-sexuality, women protest, artistic eccentricity, laziness and sadness, considered as aspects of psychopathology. Under such a vision, psychotherapy has the function of repairing the subject, or client, in order to readmit him or her into modern society, where the acquisition of a status consists in a competition between free men (sic). In this context the happy family is considered functional: fathers function as professional bread-winners, mothers as professional home-makers (Dizard and Gadlin, 1992).

The old idea of social systems as perfect systems containing sub-systems, which perfectly fit within a society of a mysterious *longa manus*, which re-equilibrate everything, is coming back in systemic therapy. Sixty years ago, Betty Friedan denounced all the premises of Ego-psychology writing the book *The Feminine Mystique* (Friedan, 2010). The book was an investigation among middle-class women belonging to the "functional family". Friedan describes women who spend their time crying on the living room sofa; when asked why they are crying, they do not know. They have all the domestic services, a good house, children going to school, a Jacuzzi and swimming pool in the garden, two cars; nevertheless, there is something that does not work in their lives, some existential dis-satisfaction. The name given by Friedan to this disease is, as in the title: "feminine mystique", a disease that has no name. The feminist movement discovered a kind of "over-determination" within the mothers and wives of the American functional world. This investigation opened the protests of the 1960s and 1970s toward the "minimal family" (Dizard and Gadlin, 1992) and a wide critique of institutionalized therapies, either behaviorist or psychoanalytical.

The Book

This book discusses theory and "clinical cases" in a way that connects ethics and aesthetics. We will deal with three main authors – Gregory Bateson, Michel Foucault and Gilles Deleuze – as well as others who have a connection to them such as Felix Guattari, Humberto Maturana, Heinz von Foerster and Francisco Varela, and yet others who have been inspired by them. In our psychotherapeutic work the most important influence is the legacy of the Milan Approach in the figures of Luigi Boscolo and Gianfranco Cecchin. Nevertheless, we are also impressed by some of the lines of social psychiatry, particularly the Italian Franco Basaglia and the Englishman Ronald Laing (1961) just to mention the most famous names. We also refer to Bateson's origin in social anthropology and to social anthropologists inspired by him and who are working with similar purposes. We put "clinical cases" in inverted commas because we are not satisfied by such an expression, as well as with expressions such as "diagnosis", "life script" or even "narrative". All these words have in common a division between the subject who enunciates – the expert clinician, diagnostician, author – and the subject of enunciation – patient, client, hero – a kind of separation between me and her/him – as in third person reporting. On the other hand, we are also dissatisfied with the idea of reducing our accounts to something that comes out from the other, even when we ask the patient to write their own version of what was going on in therapy, in the belief that this is the genuine account of the "client". In general, "clients'" accounts seem to us more adulation of the capability of the therapist, or descriptions of the miracle moment in which the client has an insight, which changes her/his life forever, than a picture or description of a complex entanglement of forces.

Any of these current positions exits in a kind of tautological position such as "tails I win, heads you lose", as for example: "Dialogic practice is a dialogic practice, then it is good because it is dialogic", or, in the opposite case: "I told her 'this' and she had an insight that was changing her life! Isn't that so, madam?" "Yes, you have completely changed my life doctor!" At the same time, we are critical of evidence-based practice (EBP). Psychotherapy cannot be reduced to a medical intervention; randomized experiments depending on diagnoses which can be unhelpful or sometimes dangerous for psychotherapy. Indeed, if biological variables are relatively stable, mental affections are constantly flowing and vanishing. If psychology is a science, it is a kind of peculiar science, which involves cultural issues, arts, literature and other issues (Barbetta, 2019; Nichterlein and Morss, 2017). Briefly we see psychology as a cultural science and psychotherapy as an applied art, which requires much more sensitiveness toward shades and nuances than toward statistic competences. This is the reason why we consider therapy as a complex art that needs a qualitative research methodology. In view of the critiques of the above methods – the holistic and the EBP – our problem is how to deal with accountability. How to give voice to people (individuals, groups, families, asylum seekers, refugees, women, disabled people, etc.) who attends therapy in a way that can be considered accountable – which does not mean how good/how bad the therapy might be, or how magic or fashionable the therapist might be. For example: put the family in a position of commenting on some raw conversational exchange after the session, reviewing the session without the presence of the therapists and vice versa, and then make the therapists listen to the comment of the family, to observe whether the comments of the family could be surprising or not from the point of view of the therapists. A practice like this, named "indefinite triangulation" (Knorr Cetina and Cicourel, 2014), assesses the rigidity of the therapist, instead of assessing the rigidity of the family, as usually happens. This could be a line of flight (Deleuze and Guattari, 1987) from the usual "double bind" of being either the expert practitioner – who reports the "clinical case" in an objective way – or the "real doctor" who collects the "needs" of a supposed client who, being "the expert", has the "privilege" of talking about him/herself, with a voice which is supposed to be subjected to the "desire of the analyst". In order to create a line of flight from such a double bind, we think we need style.

Style

What is style? The idea of "free indirect discourse" in literature (Pasolini, 1988) and "free subjective image" in cinema (1986) can help us to clarify our position.

Style has to do with the assemblage of these three components: heteroglossia, timing and nearness. For Bakhtin (1983), for example, it is not the simple idea of polyphony that matters, the phonic aspect is not just multiplied. More than a multiplication, it is an assemblage of dissonances, which, when sounding together, create an accord. In therapy, we do not speak the same language, even when we are talking the same idiom, with the same accent. Any subject – the therapists, as well as the people who attend the session – is, contemporarily, "the subject who enunciates and the subject of enunciation", as they say in literature theory. Any Otherness – including the Otherness who belongs to myself – is contemporarily a subjective and objective genitive. In an example from Joyce's "Mother's Love": it is not just the mother's love of the child, or even the child's love of the mother. Love is a time in-between the two parts, "subjective and objective genitive" (Joyce, 1922).

Nevertheless, there is a permanent gap in the languaging (Maturana and Varela, 1980) of the Otherness. For Pasolini (1988) style consists in the nearness between the author and the so-called "character", which, in style, is no longer a character in the traditional sense, but a "person" or a subject acquainted with multiple expressions, endowed with a body, which constantly interacts, languaging in singular processes not reducible to categories (Maturana and Varela, 1980; Pasolini, 1988). If the author cannot speak the idiom of the Person who inhabits the Novel, because there is a constitutive difference, nevertheless the author can be just one step nearer to the Person.

What does this mean in a book concerning therapy? Therapists, as writers, are in an asymmetric position from the very beginning of the therapeutic process. As writers, they need to find their style to be as near as possible to the persons who attend therapy, in such a way that, at the end of the process, the asymmetry has been reversed. Giving voice to the other – the character, the client, the patient – is a process of liberation from the narrative structure of the *fabula*, which, in the psy world, can mean a variety of transcendental issues: from diagnosis, to family hierarchy or dynamics. We need to find a line of flight from both diagnosis and familism.

The Collective as a Style

With our co-authorship we aim to indicate a collective who are yet not a group, who do not share a certain body of ideas or thoughts, but whose ideas and thoughts overlap, sometimes contiguously, at times touch, at times enunciate and sometimes coincide. We are not a group with a boundary, nor do we adhere to a frame of ideas within a defined set of assumptions. We are distinguished by and in our differences and we expect gaps and distances to be travelled such as has been the case in the writing of this book. We have adopted the collective as a style. Britt's anthropological sensitivity approaches Maria Esther's search for premises for getting close to children. Her approach is enunciated by Pietro's outing of psychiatric practice and categories as well as by Umberta's presentation of the clinic as a self-fulfilling prophecy. She is also insistent on the different perspectives cross-cultural contemplation can offer.

Pietro, as is the case with Umberta, has been involved with the Milan Approach since he was young. He frequently changes and revises his ideas. In this way he demonstrates affinity with the Milan group because this group changes ideas as frequently as him. Pietro admires Britt's studies on Bateson, she realized that family therapists already in the cradle have exchanged Bateson for Palo Alto. He is enchanted by Maria Esther's clinical discovering that children are revolutionary beings, or, better, revolutionary becomings. Umberta has been a student of Heinz von Foerster and found out soon that Bateson, Varela, Maturana and von Foerster are never ending masters, to be studied and re-studied, read and re-read over and over. When she found out her friend Pietro and two of his friends were talking about the clinical influence of Deleuze, she joined in with curiosity and found out that the masters are very compatible with one another. She became curious about the subtle differences and passionate about the discussions we all had together. For Maria Esther it is vital that we come from different places, along different paths, and that we speak different languages... Britt suggests we look for the difference in and through culture. Pietro invites us to go beyond the familiar to delve into those systems that breed the monsters of madness. Umberta emphasizes the need to bring back intuition and improvisation to their proper place as responsible action in an indeterminate world. Maria Esther seeks to find in childhood those revolutionary forces that transform symptoms to create new worlds. In systemic thinking revisited, each of us, all of us, have shared in the quest to regain those insights in systemic thinking which we have missed in worn-out "strategies" and "conversations".

The Chapters

Chapter 2, "Two Regimes of Madness in Psychotherapy", by Pietro Barbetta, struggles with the differences between meaning, sense and expression. It addresses the capability of the therapist to find traces in relation to the expression of what Pietro calls "deliria", in the plural. The logic of sense does not necessarily fit with the logic of meaning; the logic of sense, instead of converging in one diagnosis, gives rise to series, a proliferation of perspectives. Pietro presents a clinical series of clinical series, exploring with the reader the multiplicity of points of view to which a singularity can give rise, what Maturana and Varela (1980) would call viability.

Chapter 3, "Revolutionary Childhood", by Maria Esther Cavagnis, director of Famila y Parejas in Buenos Aires – presents a critical reflection on the dominant way of exercising the children's clinic as a captive practice and oppression of child power. The approach offers help to free the practice from its entrapment and constraints to enable life to express itself. Towards that end, a review is undertaken of current assumptions on three different dimensions: nature and culture; the family and the familiar; the story – the therapist and the child in conversation, the child as "consultant to the consultant". An attempt is made to create pathways in the clinic characterized by their revolutionary potency, and map out trajectories, thus enabling the exploration of possible new worlds.

In Chapter 4, "Thoughts from the Outside" Inga-Britt Krause, Anthropologist and Systemic Psychotherapist at the Tavistock Clinic, remembers how Gregory Bateson's ideas have been widely misunderstood by the field of family therapists starting from the beginning during the 1950s. Britt argues that a much closer understanding of Bateson must be located in France, particularly with Gilles Deleuze and Felix Guattari. In general, the cultural poverty in family therapy has led to ignorance of the relevance of anthropological investigations such as Naven, the work in Bali with Margaret Mead, and other more contemporary works. Family therapists, who declare to be Batesonian, tend not to know about the familiar kinship lexicon of the anthropological field and how this can be put to use in thinking about families, multiple positions and partial connections in therapeutic work. To this end Britt reads family positions through the work of Viveiros de Castro and Marilyn Strathern, inspired by Lévi-Strauss, Gilles Deleuze and Felix Guattari.

Chapter 5, "Getting Sick from Psychotherapy: Our Co-Responsibility in Unintended and Undesired Outcomes" is Umberta Telfener's chapter. She writes of unintended outcomes and the risk of iatrogenic risk; those nearly inevitable situations in which the worsening of the process derives from the therapeutic dance, not from the symptomatology or the personality of the client. During the last 30 years, there has in some way been an increasing fascination with the lemma "naïve therapist", as if therapists do not have skills for managing therapy. The good protest towards the authoritarianism in psychotherapy is widely confused with a naïve attitude to "everything goes". This shows the ignorance of both positions: the strategic/authoritarian one as well as the "collaborative practice" one. It is not a matter of taking a middle position, rather it is necessary to take into account other thinkers traditionally considered in the field of the systemic approach – Maturana, von Foerster, Varela, Keeney, Morin and others – as well as thinkers not considered "systemic", who created ideas which add different perspectives: Foucault, Deleuze and Guattari, de Landa, Latour, de Castro, Stiegler and many others.

In Chapter 6, "Aesthetics, Ethics and Politics in Childhood Matters", Maria Esther Cavagnis and Inga-Britt Krause consider the opportunities, when working with children, for recognizing, emphasizing and furthering innovation, the unexpected and the new. They argue that the structural functionalist mold of traditional family therapy forces children into normative ethnocentric patterns fitting with Western capitalist socio-economic structures and that the practice of child mental health professionals also tends to promote such points of view. They argue that "reality" is an effect and as such an emergence of relationships and practices and they use cross-cultural examples to develop this point. Citing research from many societies Maria Esther and Britt show that attachment may involve a multiplicity of relationships, interpretations and opportunities pointing to the complexity of the process of subjectivation. They argue for the usefulness of Foucault's notion of "the fold" in this process. They suggest that an analysis of subjectivation requires a theory of multiplicity in relationships, of partial connections, and an appreciation of "what lies behind".

Chapter 7, "Clinical Practice as Ecological Aesthetics", is written by all the authors. This was not easy to write, but probably is the chapter that clarifies many aspects of our ideas and which we had to discuss with each other again and again. From these continuous meetings and discussions a fruitful argument emerged. For instance, the insistence of Pietro on using the lemma "theory of complexity", which the other authors did not like, was helpful to find a lemma more intriguing and viable for us, "aesthetic of complexity", which further strengthened the connection between aesthetic and ethics. An ethic, which is connected with the beauty of the Earth, as in Spinoza (1677/ 2014; see also Deleuze, 1990): *Natura Naturans, Natura Naturata*, i.e. *Deus sive Natura*. An ethic that does not respond to abstract and transcendent "values", imposed by authorities from outside. No matter about religious or traditional beliefs, which may not belong to any one of us. Within the practice of psychotherapy, our main emphasis is on the admiration and respect of the beauty of life, as in the words of the poet for the stereotypical *man of science*: a primrose is nothing more than an object to be included into the Porfirian tree. Nonetheless, for the artist, there is something more. Is psychotherapy a kind of art (Barbetta, 2019; Nichterlein and Morrs, 2017)? Or is it a sui generis science? Or both?

In Chapter 8, "Babel, Bebel and Other Dangerous Glossolalia", our different preoccupations are offered as different ways of approaching ethics and aesthetics in our therapy work, in our thinking and in our engagement with each other. This chapter can then be read as so many different paths into and away from our collaboration with each other and with our other interlocutors. Maria Esther questions the standard and tired old questions in psychotherapy, such as questions about the beginning and the end, and replaces these with the question: "How does it work?" Towards the end of the chapter, she summarizes the salient points for praxis. Pietro proposes different aspects of complexity, all of which touch on and are relevant to clinical praxis. Emergence, interdisciplinarity, heterogenesis, the unconscious as a working machine, singularity, perspectivism as well as others are different ways of talking and thinking about complexity, all pointing in different directions, but also all paying attention to the question of "how does it work". Britt points out that there is no beginning and that Bateson was ahead of his time in anticipating what has been referred to as the Ontological Turn. She argues that the Ontological Turn takes difference seriously and questions some of our most embedded Western assumptions about the unified person and subject, drawing on the work of social anthropologists such as Marily Strathern, Eduardo Viveiros de Castro and Roy Wagner. This work refers to fractals, to multiplicities and to the necessity of continuously wondering and questioning both certainty and relativism. Umberta picks this up in her discussion of a clinical example and shows how in her therapeutic work she patiently aims to refrain from proposing a beginning or an end and to stay close to the unfolding profess of the therapy, working on the presence of herself and her client.

The Postscript is "The last scene of all, [...] mere oblivion" (Shakespeare, *As You Like It*, "All the World's a Stage", Jacques' soliloquy). It is the end of this eventful book and celebrates a long history of encounters, discussions, conversations and struggles.

Conclusion

We would like to stress the political praxis of this book, which may, to a superficial reading, not be easy to find because it belongs to the particular minutes of the texture concerning the clinical cases (or "series", as one of us likes to use). The corporeal turn deals with the human rights within the fields of psychiatry, asylum seekers and refugees, open discrimination against Otherness of any kind, but particularly the soft discrimination coming from the evidence of males in the chief position in families, organization, cultural clubs, hospitals, universities. Even in the dominion of psychotherapy, almost nobody has taken seriously the politics of oppression, including in sanitizing language. We think that the politics of "sanitizing language", which apparently seems to be "liberal" and respectful, could easily become an Orwellian "Newspeak".

We are used to meeting with poor people during our practice and thinking, people who speak different languages, with different accents and different dialects, with different outlooks and communications of different habitats. Nonetheless we never think of anybody as ignorant. To the contrary, we think every person belongs to their tradition, which sometimes has the hard aspect of being violent, aggressive and uncaring. Nonetheless we are confident that a good therapist possesses all the capabilities to maintain a good conversation with anyone who attends therapy, the language of respect and tenderness. The endeavor of therapy is to make a hyperbolic jump, the one suggested by Derrida (2012) in his last text on "forgiving the unforgivable, prescribe the imprescriptible". This is the way of taking a position within therapy (Foucault, 1971b).

Note

1 See also Krause's Chapter 4 of this book.

References

Bakhtin, M.M. (1983). *The Dialogic Imagination: Four Essays*. Austin, TX: University of Texas.

Barbetta, P. (2019). Percepts, affects and desire. In M. Nichterlein (ed.), *Putting the Deleuzian Machine at Work in Psychology. Annual Review of Critical Psychology*. Issue 14, pp. 153–167. www.criticalinstitute.org/journals/arcp/9

Bateson, G. (1958). *Naven: The Culture of the Iatmul People of New Guinea as Revealed through a Study of the "Naven" Ceremonial*. London: Wildwood House.

Bateson, G. (1979). *Mind and Nature: A Necessary Unity* (Advances in Systems Theory, Complexity, and the Human Sciences). New York: Hampton Press.

Blanchot, M. (1987). Michel Foucault as I imagine him. In *Foucault/Blanchot*. New York: Zone Books.

Boscolo, L., Cecchin, G., Hoffmann, L. and Penn, P. (1987). *Milan Systemic Family Therapy*. New York: Basic Books.

Cecchin, G. (1987). Hypothesising, circularity, and neutrality revisited: An invitation to curiosity. *Family Process*, 26, 405–414.

Cecchin, G., Barbetta, P. and Toffanetti, D. (2005). Who was von Foerster, anyway? *Kybernetes: The International Journal of Systems & Cybernetics*, 34(3/4), 330–342.

Deleuze, G. (1986). *Cinema 1: The Movement-Image*. Minneapolis, MN: University of Minnesota Press.

Deleuze, G. (1990). *What Can a Body Do? Expressionism in Philosophy: Spinoza*. New York: Zone Books.

Deleuze, G. (2014). *Deleuze Meets Bateson*. www.youtube.com/watch?v=6mV0bahGeOk

Deleuze, G. and Guattari, F. (1984). *Anti-Oedipus*. London: Continuing International Publishing Group (First published 1974).

Deleuze, G. and Guattari, F. (1987). *A Thousand Plateaus: Capitalism and Schizophrenia*. Minneapolis, MN: University of Minnesota Press.

Derrida, J. (2012). *Pardonner. L'imperdonable et l'imprescritible*. Paris: Galilée.

Dizard, J. and Gadlin, H. (1992). *The Minimal Family*. Amherst, MA: Massachusetts University Press.

Foucault, M. (1971a). *L'Ordre du discours*. Paris: Gallimard.

Foucault, M. (1971b). *Nietzsche, la généalogie, l'histoire: Hommage a Jean Hypplite*. Paris: PUF.

Foucault, M. (2001). *The Order of Things*. London: Routledge.

Friedan, B. (2010). *The Feminine Mystique*. London: Penguin.

Joyce, J. (1922). *Ulysses*. Paris: Shakespeare and Company.

Knorr Cetina, K. and Cicourel, A. (2014). *Advances in Social Theory and Methodology*. New York: Routledge.

Laing, R.D. (1961). *The Self and Others: Further Studies on Sanity and Madness*. London: Tavistock.

Marx, K. and Engels, F. (1998). *The German Ideology?* New York: International Publisher Company.

Maturana, H. and Varela, F. (1980). *Autopoiesis and Cognition: the Realization of the Living*. New York: Springer.

Nichterlein, M. and Morrs, J. (2017). *Deleuze and Psychology*. New York: Routledge.

Nietzsche, F. (2005). *Ecce Homo*. Harmondsworth: Penguin Books (First published 1908).

Pasolini, P.P. (1988). *Heretical Empiricism*. Indianapolis, IN: Indiana University Press.

Sartre, J.P. (1943). *L'Être et le Nèant. Essai d'ontologie phénoménologique*. Paris: Gallimard.

Spinoza, B. (2014). *Ethica: Ordine Geometrico Demonstrata*. Berlin: Nabu Press (First published 1677).

Varela, F., Thomson, E. and Rosch, E. (2017) *The Embodied Mind*. Cambridge, MA: MIT Press.

von Foerster, H. (1995). Constructions of the mind: Artificial intelligence and the humanities. *Stanford Humanities Review*, 4(2), 308–327.

Two Regimes of Madness in Psychotherapy

Pietro Barbetta

Introduction

In the following pages I deal with the transformation of institutional "radial delirium" – universal form – into segmental "multiple deliria" – plural form – in systemic therapy. "Delirium" (actually "delusion"), as "psychiatric category", is supposed to be something that could happen to all people, independent of their habits, religion, social practices, gender and other details connected to their own life script. I think that this is a big mistake. The purpose of this chapter is different. In using "delirium" as universal category, I need to show some common abstract names – "delirium", "God", "logic", for example – as universal issues. This premise comes from the idea that there is just one ontology and one epistemology. Systemic therapy works on the side of multiple phenomena dealing with bodies, art and literature.

In this chapter, I deal with complexity and those thinkers who took complexity as a point of view to analyze art, literature, sciences and therapy. I know it is difficult to read about this, just as it is difficult to write it. To me it is impossible to be clearer to the reader. At the same time, this chapter raises a lot of questions about issues that must be studied more and more. I hope to open a space for the reader to go directly to the therapeutic practice involved in the essay and to the texts and the oral communication arising from the authors mentioned.

Out of Frame, to the Origins: Doc Meets the Philosopher (Allegory)

When people from Abdera, in Thrace, invited Hippocrates (Lewin, 1968) to meet the raving Democritus, Hippocrates accepted to visit the Philosopher. The Doc saw shreds of animals scattered all around the garden beside the house. He also saw the Philosopher in the action of cutting animals up, as in anatomical studies. The Philosopher welcomed the Doc. Democritus was apparently looking for the biological origin of madness within animal remains: the black bile in Ancient Greek, *meláine chole*, from which

DOI: 10.4324/9780429437410-2

"melancholy" derives. Talking to Hippocrates, Democritus said that people who consider him mad are busy in the market all day long, wasting their lives, fighting and fussing over their affairs.

During this period, this notion of madness as "normality" was adopted, being used ironically, as in the popular remark: "Who are the madmen? Are they the ones who stay in asylums or us, who work all day long?" Within so-called "civilized" countries, in the Christian era, work became a moral stance starting from the ancient Fathers of Church, as with, for example, Cassian (fourth century) and the battle against acedia gave rise to the proverb "work ennobles man"; in such a phrase, nonetheless, the work of the unconscious is not contemplated.

Actually, what does Democritus' activity consist in at the very moment Hippocrates visits him? Democritus is cutting up animals to experiment with anatomy, in search of the black bile. When interviewed by the Doc, the Philosopher answers his interlocutor gently, and Hippocrates reports the discussion in the market in a letter. The Doc is trying to make sense of what the Philosopher is doing; the Doc transforms his activity into a discursive practice, a synthesis, a way out from the fragments of animal scattered in Democritus' garden, deprived of any meaning, except the delusional one of looking for the black bile.

Delusion – maybe for the first time in Western history – is given a meaning and is framed within a kind of social narrative concerning who is really mad. For the Doc, the fragments of animal scattered in the garden cannot be read as haruspicy. Nonetheless, I am suspicious of this story: Doc reduces the entire encounter to the discourse of the market, but what about complexity? Maybe the Philosopher, behind the apparent compulsive meaningless anatomy of animals, shows the philosophical part of madness: the marketplace.

When it becomes meaningful, delusion is explained as metaphor. The vehicle of the apparent nonsensical anatomy of animals becomes the tenor of wisdom against the market. At this very moment, madness becomes understandable in the Doc's discourse, which gives meaning to the mess that is being created in the Philosopher's garden. My proposal here is the following: let's get back to a respect for all the complexity which belongs to the philosophical garden.

Délire: Deliria as Phenomena of Art and Literature

De-lirare, literally, in Ancient Rome, means the event of going astray by the ploughshare from the path carved into the soil. In present times, *deliria* are gestures, in which I include speeches, that show the joy and grief of everyday life. Nevertheless, in clinical series, they can be transformed, as in Schreber's (1988) "feeling[s] of endless bliss".

Deleuze and Guattari write: "Every *délire* invests History before investing some ridiculous mommy-daddy" (Deleuze and Guattari, 2013), which means that in what Deleuze and Guattari call "delirium", they are not interested in psychogenesis. Deleuze is not searching the "cause" of *délire*. He and Guattari are describing such a phenomenon from different premises.

Radial, or paranoic, delirium is a repetition with no difference, you get it easily when you enter in a typical institution of power, in brief the *Psychiatric Power* (Foucault, 2008).

Segmental deliria are acts of creation (Barbetta, 2016), acts of joy and grief, which appear before the cut of language, they refuse the divisive cut. They are corporeal transformations, as in Schreber's becoming-woman. Many schizophrenics are God, Noah, Moses, Jesus, Mohammed, one of the Prophets, conquerors such as Alexander, Napoleon, hybrid creatures, kings, princesses or children of them, they have no gender or sex, no name, no religion or beliefs. Maybe they have all religions together. Deliria see women wolf-headed – as in a schizophrenic young man – diarrheal children shitting cream of pumpkin – as in a dream of a young woman who works in a restaurant – creature half badger, half lizard, corkscrew tied – as in Humpty Dumpty portmanteau words; segmental deliria are ways for becoming children. From now on, I will use the word "deliria", in plural form, in reference to segmental *délire* (Deleuze, 2008), and "delirium", in *universal* form, when I refer to the radial one (Deleuze, 1994, 2008), interpretative or paranoid "delirium".

Deliria neither begin, nor end, they are always going on, crossing a process of intuition (Bergson, 2012), entering into the thing in itself. This kind of empiricism is the one where the experience of the observer crosses the experience of the observed, they interweave and hybridize themselves. This experience is always relational, no matter if in literature, or with a family, as in therapy. It is not something that needs to be made meaningful, the idea of giving meaning to deliria is widely shared in the mental health field; all the models have in competition the idea of "interpreting" delusion: excess of dopamine, weakness of will, foreclosure of The-Name-of-the-Father, affective complexes, psychotic games, even a mis-interpretation of the double bind (Bateson, 2000b) theory, which eventually ends up with the anti-feminine concept of "schizophrenogenic mother".

In the process of giving meaning, one faces the invention of new fields of knowledge/power: neuro-psychoanalysis or cognitive-behavioral therapy, which use evidence-based medicine – what I would call "the market of the health care system". The magic process is the one that passes from the data to the general theory. From meaningless to meaningful, as in a juggle. Bernard Stiegler (2018) calls this trick "cognitive capitalism" or the "proletarianization of knowledge".[1] To overpass the limits of data, the psy-mainstream is urgently trying to create general theories of how people should deal with the world, *in order* to be healthy and sane. From the little findings of few data, one passes to general theories. My reluctance about this mainstream is because I believe that any general theory, any model for doing therapy, making it a rational process, as well as any new standardized test, works *in order* to transform segmental delusion into radial; it really works, but, as it were, for the worse.

Another problem we face concerning *délire* is the difference between "representation" and "presence". As in Sartre's novella *La chambre*, Eve, wife of the schizophrenic Pierre, feels the statues flying around them when they are tied in a hug. The statues fly faster and faster, they seem to crash on Pierre's and Eve's body, and just at the very last instant they curve touching the two bodies, making them feel as if they might die at any moment. But when Eve is with her parents, she talks as if this experience belongs only to Pierre who is the schizophrenic one. Eve lives in-between the two experiences of being mad and normal in relation to the difference between her parents and her husband. She speaks with metaphors with her parents and has deliria in the hug with Pierre; when she is with Pierre, they are joined, they are one system of raving, they are no longer two different subjects, they are a desiring machine. What makes the difference between metaphors and deliria is that metaphors are composed by two parts: tenor and vehicle (Richards, 1936). One part of a metaphor, called "tenor", is beneath, or hidden under the expression, the expression here is the vehicle, a mere representation. As in the typical example from Aristotle (1997), "the night of life", which means "senility", is the prototype of metaphor. The other part is the meaning of the hidden part. Metaphors are ways for giving meaning. Metaphors shift things into a kind of representational way, their purpose is to catch the interlocutor's feelings.

Deliria are not representations, they are *Real Presences* (Steiner, 1989). They say: "Man is sick because he's badly built" (Artaud, 2004), or "Life's but a walking shadow, a poor player/ That struts and frets his hour upon the stage/ And then is heard no more. It is a tale/ Told by an idiot, full of sound and fury/ Signifying nothing" (Shakespeare, *Macbeth*, Act 5, Scene 5, lines 24–28), where the brutality of the "thing" is immediately – with no mediation – present on your face as a new revelation.

You are not into the "night of life" because "life signifies nothing": the unbearable grief and joy of deliria. Deliria show that it is impossible to communicate, they are far from any form of colloquialism.[2] As in Macbeth's soliloquy, "a tale told by an idiot, signifying nothing", where "idiot" does not mean "less intelligent", but the one who sees beyond the meaning.

The psy-mainstream claims that schizophrenics do not understand metaphors. I think it is the contrary: it is the psy-mainstream world that does not understand deliria. As far as I met "schizophrenics", they do not like metaphors, a metaphor is always matter of being entangled in persuasion that they are "really mad". Deliria are real creations, declarations about something that really exists out there in the world, they are material, like scratches, casts, fragments disposed here and there in chaotic way with no conscious purpose. Deliria are disparate systems, incoherent, with no synthesis. Deliria are the making of the world, they come from the materiality of fragments embodied into life.

A real creation is, for example, Lewis Carroll's "Jabberwocky".[3] It consists in the creation of portmanteau words with no sense, which challenge the unconscious in creating images. "What are toves?" asks Alice to Humpty Dumpty, and *he/she/it* answers:

> Well, "toves" are something like badgers – they're something like lizards – and they're something like corkscrews.
>
> (Carroll, 1941, p. 116)

In the formula: "image formation processes are unconscious", Bateson (1979, 2000c) stresses an issue that psychoanalysis neglects: perception. Images are, first of all, percepts and affects (Barbetta, 2018), which are disparate and unconscious, they are syntheses of image formation, the process of extracting forms from chaos. One can imagine all men as blades of grass, moving with the wind, at the feet of Claude Monet's *Woman with a Parasol*. Such an image arises from the work of the unconscious, but if I were a very Catholic person, I would probably see the image of Maria, with a veil – no parasol – and all humanity at her feet in another kind of veneration. Same percepts, different affects. In Bateson, as well as in Deleuze and Guattari, deliria – dreams, art, poetry, imagination, movie sequences – are auto-*poietic* phenomena (Maturana and Varela, 1980), which means that deliria produce an endless production of immanent desire in a *continuous plateau of intensity* (Bateson, 2000d; Deleuze and Guattari, 1987). You are agglutinated to what you are doing.

Series, the *Téchne* of Therapy

The mainstream approach to delirium comes from outside of deliria, and reproduces the mechanism of splitting Language from bodies, as if Language (capitalized) would be transcendent from the immanence of body. In trying to connect these two parts, languages and bodies, I stress the importance of the relation between enunciation and visibility (Foucault, 2011).

Enunciation deals with discourses about something, visibility deals with observation of something (Deleuze, 2018). When one enunciates something, one deals with comments or critique; when one observes something, one deals with practice and desire. There are systems of enunciation, on which one can comment or critique – such as, for example, the Diagnostic and Statistical Manual of Mental Disorders – and systems of visibility – such as, for example, the work done in mental health institutions, and the treatments of delusional bodies – which someone practices.

One enunciates a diagnosis but observes ties on bed, hyper-administration of chemical substances, locked doors. Treatments are not declarations, they are acts, sometimes abusive: practices that satisfy authoritarian desires of oppression.

The passage from the diagnostic discourse – the criteria for a diagnosis of "delusional episode" – to the practice of medication is still, and will remain, a "scientific mystery". Tying patients on the bed is not different from other violent acts: battering women, rejecting asylum seekers, mistreating children.

Later on, in the following pages, I will write about *clinical series* where the oppression is hidden under the veil of normality, and cruelty remains undergrounded in neutral words. In using the lemma "clinical series", I recognize that it is no easy to give an immediate and clear meaning to the word "series". It is a word frequently used by Gilles Deleuze (1993b). "Series" is a fuzzy set. In series there is dissension, difference and also repetition. "Series" means that any event has multiple origins and multiple pragmatic effects.

In the language of the Milan Approach, it is possible to make a multiplicity of hypotheses concerning any event, and in the process of the event unfolding, the hypotheses change, the same as, in mathematics, the unfolding of a curve changes the direction of the tangent line instant by instant. Within the Milan Approach, "series" is the idea expressed by the statement: "Do not fall in love with your own hypotheses". For example: what happens behind the one-way mirror is different from what is going on inside the session of therapy. The inside position does not inform the outside position, the two – inside and outside – perturb each other. Any time I am going back and forth, from the therapy room to the one-way mirror space, shared by my colleagues – who observe the session from "outside" – I feel myself as an anthropologist who brings different accounts of my interior affective experience. Therapy is unstable and fluctuating. It is an affective constructivist experience (Barbetta, 2015; Boscolo, 1991; Boscolo et al., 1988; Telfener and Casadio, 2003).

The constructivist experience does not deny affective realities (ontologies); it rather stresses the multiple affections over reality (epistemology). In constructivism, affective relations are something "out there"; nevertheless, any gaze over reality comes from the point of view of the observer (von Foerster, 1982), and the observer is not just a simple subject, or a "Self"; rather the observer is a system.

Metamorphosis

As in Maturana and Varela (1980), living systems are open and closed at two different levels; while they are open in changing their structure, systems cannot change their life until they die and even later on. There are memories of what remains alive. It is the process of metamorphosis, from butterflies to frogs, things change and remain the same. The way of grasping this ontological process from the epistemological one is "perspectivism". "Perspectivism", is a good word to summarize the Milan Approach. Realities are transformed, by the points of view, in different degrees, I am unfolded within the reality I am living. Depending on the context, any reality has indefinite points of view and, although points of view are infinite, they are limited at the same time.

Ontologically, life is an infinite and senseless flux of becoming; hypotheses are points of view concerning life, finite parts of life, they provide "the sense of an ending" within life (Kermode, 2000), they are "conic perspectives" into the "cylindric life". Maybe the reader is not familiar with some geometric intuition. Let me try to clarify how geometry deals with affects: imagine a cylinder – you can draw one on paper right now – as you see, it has something of the absolute. Now, let us imagine a cone; you see that drawing it with your pen on the same paper, you can insert the cone within the cylinder. Nonetheless, within the same cylinder, you can insert not just "this cone" you drew, but an infinite number of other cones that you can draw. For example, in the way writers create novels, there is a reality out there (the cylinder). Series are immanent and in circular position to reality, as cones are immanent to the cylinder.

In his lessons on *Leibnitz and the Baroque*, Deleuze (1993a) talks about two different perspectives to the world, which he calls respectively the "cylindric" and "conic" perspective. What is the cylindric perspective? Any point of the space works as an infinity of lines that converge in the cylinder. This means also that this is the point of concurrence, at infinite, to infinite distance. As in the Euclidean space: two parallel lines have no points of convergence; they have no *cline*, points of inclination. Conic perspectives have inclination. They are points of concurrence at finite distance, what Bateson (2000c) calls "creature". It is important the mutual immanence of these two perspectives. The cylindric perspective is present in all the conic perspectives, all the conic perspectives are present in the cylindric one. It is a change of shapes: *metamorphosis*.

In a cylindric space it is possible to insert an infinite number of cones, any cone is a point of view on the cylinder. The cylinder has infinite perspectives. In constructivist terms: reality, out there, exists; it is the condition of possibility to create infinite points of view. Reality is an infinite senseless flux of becoming, but there are points of view on reality. Thinking of the inexistence of reality denies the material unfolding of things and bodies, the continuous changing of reality. At the same time, things are inserted in a process of "metamorphosis", they change their shape under different gazes.

The Importance of Anamorphosis for Series

Later on – during the lectures on Leibnitz – Deleuze (1993a) used a second, different word, besides "metamorphosis": "anamorphosis". What is the difference between "metamorphosis" and "anamorphosis"? If "metamorphosis" means the passage from one shape into another; "anamorphosis" is the passage from the inform into form – pleroma unfolds into creature – a kind of taking-form, as in generative ontogenetic processes. Is it what Gregory Bateson (2000c) calls "pleroma"? I do not have an answer for this question, nonetheless, Deleuze argues:

In appearance the whole is disorder, you do not recognize anything, everything is tangled. You have a series of inflections that go everywhere and, into this, you distinguish nothing. Well, the point of view is how to extract a shape from such a disorder. No more something that makes the passage from a form into another, but what extracts shape, whatever form, starting from the unshaped.

(Deleuze, 1975/1976, from 1:15:00 on)

Here Deleuze shows the second side of constructivism: it is not just the point of view of the subject; it is the aesthetical complexity of observing systems. Something, out there, is matched by the eye; nonetheless, to grasp it, the observer has to take position at the margins of the thing. We are facing two different points of view: 1) there is a point of view of the observing systems on realities (epistemology); 2) but there is also a point of view *inside* realities (ontology).

Realities ask to be observed from a certain point of view: the "marginal" position. When your hypothesis becomes dominant, you have to abandon it. Ontology and epistemology interact creating order from noise: anamorphosis. Realities have a place, a locus, crossed by the points of view of the observer; at the same time realities are out there in a group of transformations.

Well – Deleuze (1975/1976, 1:28:00) continues – the sun is a point of view on the planet's movement, ok. But you and me, we are points of view on the world. We are points of view on the infinite series of the world. Because any point of view is on a series... any point of view subsumes a series. What series? The series of transformation through which passes the object... The world orders itself... Nevertheless, if it is true that any point of view defines itself through series, we all are points of view on the series of the world (Deleuze, 1975/1976).

Shaping Series: Style, Chaosmosis

In literature, movie-making and other forms of art, style has to do with "series". Far from being "theory", "style" regards the way to approach Otherness. For Deleuze (1986, 1989), Bateson (2000a) and Pasolini (2005)[4] style deals with freedom, it liberates the character from scripts and plots, de-framing the subject from the slavery of narrative. Series do not concern just the subject, series are ways of describing systems and description of systems. In this sense they are not merely reports separated from clinical work, they are still part of the therapeutic process.

Pasolini uses the lemma "free indirect discourse" – a style of writing – to show how the writer approaches eventuality and singularity. Although between the writer and the character there is a constitutive difference – they belong to different worlds and different ontologies – nevertheless, the writer has to create series as close as possible to the world of the character: the character becomes no longer a character. For Pasolini, slangs, dialects, vernacular languages, different linguistic registers, idiolects are assembled to create recounts, novellas, novels, poetry, movies.

Chaosmosis (Guattari, 1995) is a complex system – of literature, music, painting, computing, therapy and so on – composed by three types of lines: molar, molecular and lines of flight. *Molar lines* are the composition taming, they are axiomatic and delineate the tradition: line of filiation, general principles of literature, formal logic, rules of painting, making music and so on; even the masters who founded the field, like the medical doctors who gave their names to diseases, the most important musical composers and so on have to obey molar lines. There is a lineage that connects molar lines in a kind of vertical way, like blood heritage, DNA transmission, logical axioms, foundational stories, masterpieces, etc. *Molecular lines* are bridges; they create connections, or alliances, between different molar lines. The molar system of bees and the molar system of flowers create reproduction; viruses – the contemporary pandemic crisis is an example – bridge different types of DNA or RNA into cells; parasitical or cooperative symbiosis bridges different organisms; the *Tetralogy of Jacob Stories*, by Thomas Mann, bridges the Hebrew *Genesis* composition with contemporary literature. Interconnections between molar and molecular create singularities, they can be observed as becoming systems of explanation. *Lines of flight* introduce hyper-complexity (Morin, 1990) into the systems; they twist axiomatic systems, or literary taming, into an upsetting disorder; they create systemic regressions, which move as far as to fragment sounds into noise, creating a different temporary order-from-noise.

Pasolini (2005) is an important point of reference in regards to the constitution of series in literature and cinema. The ability to write in *free indirect style* – or to make *subjective images* in long shooting videos – is an art of assembling together molar and molecular lines with lines of flight. I am convinced that this art is part of the therapeutic process.

When he writes about free indirect style, Pasolini (2005) means the art of being close to the idiom, the body, the expression of the character, using her proper words, gazes, faciality, as far as to take a minimal distance to the character. The *character* is no more a one-dimensional *being*, rather the character becomes a collective subject, part of her community and, at the same time, a system of becoming different from herself.

Pasolini stresses the social point of literature: the character is the inhabitant of a certain kind of social condition, which has to do with the speech used in the social environment. The character becomes persona in making a difference from her communitarian and social world. Now, if one substitutes the word "character" with the word "client", or "person who attends psychotherapy", one can easily see the art of therapy in action. Free indirect style in literature corresponds to the "subjective free image" in cinema, which is the way of showing corporeal images; this is also therapy. Deleuze explains it in these words:

> A character acts on the screen, and is assumed to see the world in a certain way. But simultaneously the camera sees him, and sees his world

from another point of view, which thinks, reflects and transforms the viewpoint of the character [...] Pasolini cites as examples Antonioni and Godard. And, indeed, Antonioni is one of the masters of obsessive framing: in it the neurotic, or the man losing his identity, enters into a "free indirect" relationship with the poetic vision of the director who affirms himself in him, through him, whilst, at the same time, distinguishing himself from him.

(Deleuze, 1986, p. 75)

This use of the camera allows Godard and Antonioni to express the instability, or the uneasiness, of being at an in-between point in French, or Italian, post-war society in transformation. The singularity of the camera experience discloses these peculiar styles of movie-making, the long shot creates intensity, you see the subjective experience from the virtual experience of yourself, intermediated by the movie-maker's style. A triadic experience: you, the character, the movie-maker all together embedded within the movie-making system. Clinical series should become the subjective free image style in psychotherapy. Series are neither clinical reports nor clinical narratives. They are rather points of view, observatories that assemble together molar and molecular lines with lines of flight. For example: describing the ability of a man in talking to dogs, admiring a wolf-woman.

Clinical Series

Perspectivism

In consequence of the distinction between deliria and metaphor I made earlier, we should distinguish "creation" from "interpretation". Interpretations come from the outside expert's gaze – the academic, the scholar, the cognitive-capitalist – who is supposed to know the matter and frames or traps creation into a making-meaningful authoritarian cognitive-behavioral-marketing machine. What I call "series" are not just stories, or cases, they neither necessarily get consistency, nor do they describe facts, as chronicles. Clinical series are rather bits of temporary hypotheses, kind of delusional supplements that show the emergence of the interweaving practice of relationships. Series are groups of transformation (Piaget, 1973), metamorphoses and creatures (Bateson, 1979).

Clinical series – rather than being clinical reports by experts – do not talk throughout the filter of clinical theories or diagnosis; they play within the imaginary world, the unconscious, as in Gaston Bachelard's idea of *rêverie* (Bachelard, 1992).

One of the key aspects of clinical series is the choice of names. Usually, in clinical cases, you have to change the name of the person, just for privacy reasons; in this case, whatever the name should be, if it is different from the real one, it is fine. Sometimes clinicians use the first letter of the name, as P., for example for Peter or Paul. Nevertheless, names have histories; Peter and Paul are different series; Peter is the owner of heaven's key, Paul is the one who converted himself on Damascus way, becoming temporarily blind. Paul is the one who wrote a lot of letters, reinterpreting the Bible to be adapted to Christianism. In other series, Peter is the guy who lives in Never-Ever-Land, Paul is the Lord who runs the Beatles. Hence these names have different lines of flight. Apparently, following the two plots I mentioned, Peter is a man of few words and no memory, who lives in an extraordinary place outside the world; Paul is a story teller, sometimes boring, who made the grade in Christianity, and at the Chamber of Lords.

Clinical series, instead of being bureaucratic control of privacy, are folds, they have a minimal distance from historical events: changes of names, jobs, gender, city, country (if any), family, ethnic group, language spoken and other details are all imaginary variants of reality. The trace that remains constant is the system of affects, the quality of relationships, the drama.

In writing about the other, I am always writing about myself, even though I am writing here, on my desk, I am in relationship to the other, in this very moment, as if I am writing her a letter. In clinical series, I am entangled in connecting stories, expressions, faciality, bodies related one to the other. In *Schizoanalysis* (Deleuze and Guattari, 2013) the series are creations and variations of name, gender, profession, political position, religious beliefs, national belonging, age, language, health, body shape and so on. These variations can neither be totally free, nor totally stuck, as different virtual realities, which, in the case of therapy is delusional pro-longation of what cannot be grasped completely. The non-oedipalized persona (Deleuze and Guattari, 2013) gets no stable name, gender, iden-tity, political, religious, ethnical position; *It* (*Id, Es*) is no more *sub-juga-ted, it* is a collection of fragments.

First Clinical Series: The Young Film-Maker

Blaise is a young film-maker, he comes from a destitute family and lives in the middle of a North Italian province, where disparity between richness and poverty is blatant; the rich people are usually building contractors, connected to criminality; the poor ones are peasants, masons or carpenters. In a place like this, people barely know standard Italian, and usually speak an incomprehensible dialect. Blaise's father – whom I name Guido – is a truck driver and his mother, Carolina, a housewife. As usually happens in these families, Carolina and Guido had two mouths to feed over the last 20 years: Blaise, the young man who sits in front of me, and his sister Camilla. Considering the environment – which seems to be a gym for young "rebels without a cause", or joining the workforce of criminal bands – unusually the two children grew up going willingly to school: particularly Blaise.

Blaise sits on a chair in front of me. From my point of view, I see his dignity and his pride at being a person who is doing everything to further his passion of becoming a film-maker. He has no money to get to the right school; it is too expensive, and I remember what trouble I also had when I was his age, working to pay for my studies.

During adolescence, Blaise attends high school in the bigger town near the village and, later on, he goes to a film-making school in Milan. Soon after he finds jobs with different television companies and becomes second director to an art director, an older woman with whom he had a romantic relationship, recently ended. Both partners dislike the ménage, and, after a couple of years, the relationship falls apart.

After few years of living this unsatisfied life, Blaise returns to the family home. He returns because his father is opposed to Camilla studying at university. Blaise feels he needs to help Camilla handle their father's "ignorant and brutal authoritarianism". Blaise describes him as a corpulent truck driver: an ignorant person who always shouts and yells when, late in the evening, he gets back home. There is always something to argue about, but Guido is not physically violent, he just screams. Blaise feels a mixture of pity and resentment towards his father, and we share the impression of a man who "took the wrong way in life", we also share the idea that Guido had no other choices. The mother always says not to bother him, that he has a lot of problems with the truck and is physically devastated by hours of driving. It seems like the scenario of Arthur Miller's *Death of a Salesman*, but, unlike Miller's drama, the two children never go astray. Guido is a truck driver and Willy Loman is a salesman. Both are driving all day long. Nevertheless, Guido works in solitude, Willy meets people. If a salesman is forced to be a *trickster*,[5] a *truck driver* is always alone, no smiles or shoe shining, he's just a biological prosthesis of his own truck.

I feel that, in coming to therapy with me, Blaise is looking for a different father, but I do not feel that Guido has been a bad father for Blaise. Guido is simply a person who was raised to be a truck driver, in a poor family, during the 1960s, in a village in northern Italy. I feel that there will be a time, a moment, or an imaginary space, where Blaise and Guido will join. I feel that I am just a wire that connects the two men, father and son, in a tender way. The moment when Blaise comes for therapy coincides with the moment when he comes back home after breaking off the affair with the older woman he met in Milan. His work at home consists in staying hours on the computer, working on the moviola, editing movies. Guido does not understand it as a "real" work. Whenever Guido comes back home, he accuses Blaise, saying: "Instead of staying all day long playing on the computer, get out and find a job!"

Blaise's work, particularly now that he is back home, is not yet so profitable.

Guido spends the time at home groaning and grumbling about almost everything. The two men, Guido and Blaise, frequently quarrel in front of the two women. Blaise tells me that being at home exhausts him, yet, at the same time, he feels he ought to stay to protect the rest of the family. Blaise sees himself as a guardian. During the period of my encounters with Blaise, Guido retired from work and Blaise's description of Guido changed. He began to describe Guido as a tired old man who spent all his life driving trucks to stay away from the toxic environment of the village and the community where they live: a poor, tired old man, as in Arthur Miller's final part of *Death of a Salesman*, but with no redemption even when he dies.

In one of the sessions, I ask Blaise where he would like to live, how he could turn his gaze on his passion and desire, and what would happen to "take this road for his life".

Now Blaise shows another part of himself: starting from the moment he returned home from Milan, he looks for a new advanced film-making course abroad. The one in Milan is enough for working on television broadcasts, although he wants to be a real film-maker. After research online, Blaise finds an important school in London for what he needs, but it is too expensive. Then he finds another school in Edinburgh, much cheaper. Experts say that this school is even better than the London one, but it is very difficult to get a position. As part of the application process, one has to send a short movie to the assessors.

After a few encounters – talking again and again about his father, and Blaise's divided feelings towards him – Blaise decides to apply to Edinburgh. He thinks that the only hope of being admitted at such a school lies in making a movie about his father: "A big challenge!" I say, "With my father as the interpreter of himself", he says. The first time he has such an idea during the encounters, he makes as if to rise from the sofa, lifts his head and looks directly into my eyes: "Yes" he says, "this is a very good idea!", pointing his finger at me, as if identifying me as the author of the idea of filming Guido: an idea which, in fact, came from himself.

During the following meetings the therapy room becomes a workshop for designing the way of making his father an interpreter of himself. At home, the father accepts the part, and the two men of the family start to collaborate for the first time. Not easy at all! When Blaise gives instructions to Guido, he acts in a very naïve and childish way, making the two women in the family laugh. Blaise, unsatisfied and disappointed, day by day, becomes agitated over how Guido is being wimpish and dull. Blaise starts to scream, scolding his father as if the asymmetry between the two has totally reversed. Guido starts to answer as usual: "I am not used to being scolded by anyone, particularly by my child. Is that clear enough!?" and the machine records Guido's reaction to Blaise. The two women understand that Guido's reaction is working for the movie, so they also start to provoke Guido again and again, provoking Guido's rebellion, and the machine continues to record everything. The movie is ready in a few weeks. During this period nobody tells Guido that the movie is going well; all family members maintain a moody and resentful attitude towards Guido, as if they were really angry. After a few days, Guido goes to Blaise, saying: "Look, I don't think this idea of making the movie with me is a good one. After all I am just a driver. I have no skills, and now that I'm retired, I won't continue this way". "Don't worry", says Blaise, "the movie is finished; it is a series of long shots of you". And Guido says, "Speak clearly, what do you mean?" Blaise says, "I'll show you". Blaise was able to introduce the camera into the real world of his family, using the real person as an interpreter of himself, as in Jonathan Caouette's movie *Tarnation*.[6]

My impression concerning Blaise's therapy is that I did relatively little. The main thing I achieved was to feel a resonance between my life and Blaise's. I had been in Blaise's position 40 years earlier, when I was in my twenties. The difference is that I did not have a father like Blaise's, although I also struggled to study and become who I am now. I had to work and stop my studies, then restart, when I had the money to continue. In certain moments, when Blaise was coming to me, I felt as if I were a second, temporary father for him. When he became capable of changing his affections toward Guido, it was time for me to retire my temporary feelings. Blaise went to Scotland, and I hope he had the possibility of progressing in his desire to become a movie-maker, or whatever he hoped to be.

As you see, in the above account, the most important thing has been the affect of having had a similar experience when I was in the same period of life as Blaise. I never told him about my life, but nonetheless, it was as if Blaise and I shared a similar experience in the realm of the unconscious: a meta-morphosis from my form of life, when I was 20, into a real presence of himself.

Second Clinical Series: The Man Who Talks with Dogs

This is the first story I heard concerning Ambleto, recounted by his parents:

Ambleto is a young man who lives with his family: his father, Claude, his mother Lisbeth, his sister Ortensia and two dogs. He is doing very well at school until he is 18, when he starts to talk only to the two dogs belonging to the family. At the same time, he maintains less and less contact with the human family members, reducing his language to a few barks. While he loses the conversational language with people, his glossolalia with the dogs improves, and the dogs seem to consider Ambleto part of their own "people". Time goes by and the situation consolidates increasingly in terms of Amble-to's self-exclusion from the human enclave. It is as if he is transforming him-self into a dog, and even his body seems to change.

One day, Claude brings Ambleto to the emergency psychiatric unit. Ambleto refuses to be admitted to hospital and after being forced to remain for some days and take anti-psychotic medication, he becomes passive. Dis-missed by the hospital, he returns home and, at the very moment when Claude goes to pick Ambleto up to take him home, a nurse, or MD, whispers in Claud's ears: "your son has a severe psychosis, you had better put medi-cation secretly in his food". Following these whispers, a radial delirium spreads out from the utterance whispered to Claude. After being dismissed by the hospital, the young man becomes more and more aggressive towards his family members, banging doors and furniture and breaking objects. Even the dogs are now terrorized by Ambleto's violence and protests. The dogs start to avoid Ambleto, and he becomes more and more isolated within the family and amongst friends. Even if the hospital's advice to administer medication in his food has apparently remained a secret, from this moment on Ambleto begins to accuse his family of poisoning his food. He refuses to eat. It is as if he had met the Ghost of the "Real Father" who told him: "Look, someone put a *leperous distilment* in your father's ears!"

When returning home, Claude – a strong farmer who works all day long – starts to master the child. Nonetheless, during the most of the day, Claude is outside and the two women face Ambleto's hostility. Particularly Ortensia, who often remains shut up in her room, fearful of her brother's threats.

Although she feels love towards her brother, Ortensia starts to fast and becomes thinner and fearful. Now both, Ambleto and Ortensia are losing weight, becoming more and more thin. After the psychiatric hospitalization, Ambleto refuses to go to any kind of psychotherapy, or counselling, and Ortensia, who witnesses the worsening of Ambleto after hospitalization, also refuses to go to therapy. The parents think that Ortensia, having witnessed what happened after Ambleto had been held in psychiatric unit, does not want to deal with psy-people. After a period of paranoia, Ambleto, whose parents refused to give him medication, alternates moments when he is going to work with the father, with moments when he feels himself confused, as if his brain were clogging up.

This is the account given me by Ambleto's parents during the few meetings we had, without the two children, who both refused to attend therapy. I still have in mind the expression of these two persons. They appeared desperate to me, as if, after Ambleto's psychiatric hospitalization, they did not see any way out of the "illness of our family", as Lisbeth says. After a few sessions with the two parents, Ambleto agrees to meet Doctor Polino, a therapist and MD. Polino is congenial enough to become acceptable to Ambleto, and they start a kind of comedy therapy:

What do you read, my lord?
Words, words, words.

Third Clinical Series: The Wolf-Woman – Ortensia in Therapy

I and Ambleto's parents decided to suspend family therapy temporarily, awaiting what might happen during the meetings of Polino and Ambleto. A few months later Ortensia, Ambleto's sister, called me. The moment when Ortensia comes to therapy coincides with the changes in Ambleto's attitude of being aggressive towards her. However, she is still fearful and sad for what happened to her brother and family. During our encounters, Ortensia finishes her university studies, finds a job, then another one, and another; and she is able to find them with no periods of unemployment, although she never experiences any job satisfaction. Finally, she finds a new job in the big city, 40 miles from the family home. Going back and forth is hard, but she does not want to leave her parents alone with Ambleto. She is still worried about her brother's possible reactions. Attending therapy, Ortensia is apparently improving. Ortensia is a beautiful young woman, I am totally surprised to see a cultivated young lady, who seems to come from a noble family, completely different from the style of her parents. The previous symptoms of fear and sadness are less vivid and she is gaining weight, becoming more and more beautiful.

In a few months, Ortensia meets a man in the big city: Fausto, ten years older than her. The man falls in love with her and quite soon they move in together.

Fausto is going to be more and more attracted by her and demands more sexual encounters. During this period, Ortensia presents the difficulty of having sexual intercourse with Fausto, and nightmares. Within a few months, the relationship with Fausto starts to become critical, and I feel that I am not able to establish a viable resonance with her. I start to think in terms of the usual mainstream of family therapy: "anorexia necessitates family therapy", I feel myself trapped by a stubborn and repetitive hypothesis, arising from systemic handbooks.

Ortensia feels that her corporeal transformation expresses the anger of having been physically abused by her brother; she also remembers being sexually abused when she was 18 by a 40 year old man. Ortensia tells me that maybe she is going to punish Fausto to prevent the sudden transformation of him into Ambleto or into the previous abuser when she was 18. The three become one, as in radial delirium. And I am also a man, so what should I do? Should I refer her to a woman therapist? Maybe in family therapy? When I experience these affects, the sessions change their direction. Ortensia is convinced that she is going to become a wolf, which terrorizes Fausto. She confesses that she would recover sexual pleasure if she could become a kind of executioner woman for Fausto. But, she says, Fausto has no notion of entering a kind of masochistic relationship. He is the typical Italian "good family boy". Fausto might be scared by Ortensia's "perverted" desire, as she says. I am on the point of ending our meetings; I feel Ortensia needs a woman to continue in this way. At the same time, I am also concerned with her transformation, and I am curious about a kind of replication of Ambleto's symptoms in Ortensia. Discussing this with colleagues, I decide to not interrupt the therapy. I feel that my curiosity is going to resonate with her body changes. During this period of therapy, Ortensia has recurrent dreams, more or less the same: she dreams about a monster, a persecutor who terrorizes her. The monster takes different shapes in different dreams and tries to kill her. She flees from the threat, running here and there, but when she finds a safe place, the persecutor reappears, and she runs away again, forever and ever, until she wakes up.

For a period, therapy seems to be at a sticking point. During the same period she goes back and forth to find her brother, because Ambleto is also going back and forth from the psychiatric unit. Now Ortensia has a mixture of dreams: sometimes she dreams of me, trying to calm her, sometimes she dreams of the monster, which terrorizes her. Am I both the characters of her dreams? The relationship with Fausto is almost over and she also feels abandoned; Ortensia says that she is dreaming of my presence in her life as the only one who is taking care of her. I am worried about her condition during those days, even though she has physically recovered. I tell her to call me whenever she feels uncomfortable with herself; probably I am seeing her as the daughter I never had. One of those days, she brings a different dream to therapy:

I am in my parents' home, as if I never left it; as during the period of university, when I was traveling back and forth so as not to leave my parents alone with Ambleto. I carry a tiny dog in my arms and I know that there is a big wolf in my room, ferocious because she has been starving for many days. My parents are forcing me to enter. My mother pushes me into the room and closes the door behind me, with the puppy dog in my arms. The wolf is on my bed and she is worse than I could have imagined; indeed, she has long spears all around her body. I try to escape, but the room is tiny, so the wolf will savage me. But instead, she comes very close and I realize that the wolf has no spears on her head. She is looking for tenderness, and I caress her head. The dream ends and I feel free of my usual anxiety and joyful after dreaming. At this very moment, I get the feeling I want to talk to dogs, that there is nothing wrong with this! Fausto has a dog and I'll start to talk to her! I'd like to show Ambleto that now I speak to dogs, as he used to do before the hospitalization.

Conclusions

My intention in this chapter was to show deliria as a particular kind of aesthetic and ethic experience. Artaud, Carroll, Shakespeare and all the other creators I mentioned – including the talking-man-dog, the film-maker, the wolf-woman – form series. Life-series: the unfolding scripts of people who I met in my clinical experience from the end of the 1980s until now, during the last 35 years of clinical work with other colleagues within the systemic field as it has been shaped and conceived in Milan. I did my best to assemble parts of clinical work, literary fragments, memories of what I learned during my life and my therapeutic curiosity. The question I pose in this essay is: how far we can go in "giving meaning" to deliria? Has meaning noise, or sound? Do connections between noise and sound, as in glossolalia, have meaning? Has the man who passed the night in conversation with a talking sex-machine a meaning? Or the other one, who is in love with the neighbor's dog?

Giving meaning means to explain delusion; the work I propose in therapeutic conversation is to continue it, to add other deliria to deliria and to re-open the universal radial delirium to the multiplicity of deliria, as when the film-maker found a way to welcome his truck-driver father as an actor, or when Ortensia came back to the canine practice of talking with dogs – all this passes through tenderness, not awareness.

Unfortunately, many clinical theories and institutional practices teach psychiatrists, social workers, nurses and psychologists to transform segmental polyphonic deliria into monolingual paranoid delirium and instructions to get rid of it. The way of presenting a clinical case – immediately transforming deliria into symptoms (Foucault, 1964) – is the *punctum* of this chapter.

Every transformation of deliria into delirium is the "condition of possibility" for the existence of psychiatry as a discipline, in the two senses of knowledge and subjugation. Clinical practices widely share the idea that deliria are severe symptoms, incurable and sometimes dangerous, no matter if – as in the DSM or the ICD – all criteria of defining delusion change time by time, and clinician by clinician. Nonetheless, deliria, in their plural version and uncanny content, scare the psy-mainstream. Reactions and threats of seclusion still belong to the psy-mainstream field.

In the field of psychology, the mainstream shares the idea of making the "patients/clients" aware of what "they" do. In my view, awareness is nothing, but gives meaning of something going on in a – Joycean – *stream of consciousness*. If you look at the terminology of the psy-mainstream discourse: *mental disorder* must be cured *in order to* be successful, make the grade, being productive, bear an obedient body, "accepting" injustice, unfair authoritarian relationships or harassment at work, arrogance on the street, violence at home, poverty, women's submission to men, children's violation, etc.

It is not just the simple operation done by the single clinician; it is rather a process of transformation of deliria based on diagnostic practices and the consequent treatment, as if mental affections would be medical diseases. The "unaware patients" often do not claim to be ill and refuse to be treated. The "patients" start to be paranoid because there is a real process of persecution, which consists in the practice of forcing them to admit their illness (Foucault, 2008). Differently from other branches of medicine, in mental health, the institution does not recognize the right to refuse the cure, so "cure" easily turns into "perpetration", as in the case of the young man who talks to dogs.

Clinical series are just one step closer to the event, although they are not the mere repetition of it, they are not what really happens, they are other series which go in parallel with reality out there. The event in therapy is the repetition of the real event, with differences; it is the event in a group of transformations. In Milan systemic therapy, we share the idea that grief comes essentially from not being listened to and not being observed by others – grief is an issue of communication.

To be disconfirmed by your relatives, precious friends, colleagues, medical doctors and psychologists makes things worse. I know there is grief in deliria, but the main grief belongs to the imposed remedies. This is the reason for the Milan Approach to family therapy to recognize human rights for "mad" people. What usually happens at the hospital is the reverse: if once, in your family, you were weird and strange, now at the hospital you do not exist anymore, you are part of a paranoid delusional system; they call such a process a "cure". Bateson (2000e) calls this kind of discursive practice "pathologies of epistemology": authoritarian practices, veiled by a supposed medical treatment.

We deal not with a single syndrome but with a genus of syndromes, most of which are not conventionally regarded as pathological. Let me coin the word "transcontextual" as a general term for this genus of syndromes. It seems that both those whose life is enriched by transcontextual gifts and those who are impoverished by transcontextual confusions are alike in one respect: for them there is always or often a "double take". A falling leaf, the greeting of a friend, or a "primrose by the river's brim" is not "just that and nothing more". Exogenous experience may be framed in the contexts of dream, and internal thought may be projected into the contexts of the external world. And so on (Bateson, 2000e, p. 277).

Notes

1 Stiegler uses the lemma "proletarianization of knowledge" for describing the limited technological knowledge of the researcher, when Marx describes the proletarian as the subject who knows just the limited part of an engine, that must be assembled in the whole of the machine, he mentions the fact that the proletarian has to create a perfect part of such a machine, but knows nothing about the whole. The same thing happens to the researcher at the present time.
2 Roman Jakobson makes this claim, analyzing the conversations with other people during the very last days of the schizophrenic poet Hölderlin (Jakobson, 1986); far from any form of colloquialism, Hölderlin created the most beautiful poetry of his life: *Die Aussicht* (*The Perspective*).
3

'Twas brillig, and the slithy toves
Did gyre and gimble in the wabe:
All mimsy were the borogoves,
And the mome raths outgrabe.

Beware the Jabberwock, my son!
The jaws that bite, the claws that catch!
Beware the Jubjub bird, and shun
The frumious Bandersnatch!"

He took his vorpal sword in hand;
Long time the manxome foe he sought –
So rested he by the Tumtum tree
And stood awhile in thought.

And, as in uffish thought he stood,
The Jabberwock, with eyes of flame,
Came whiffling through the tulgey wood,
And burbled as it came!

One, two! One, two! And through and through
The vorpal blade went snicker-snack!
He left it dead, and with its head
He went galumphing back.

And hast thou slain the Jabberwock?
Come to my arms, my beamish boy!
O frabjous day! Callooh! Callay!
He chortled in his joy.

'Twas brillig, and the slithy toves
Did gyre and gimble in the wabe:
All mimsy were the borogoves,
And the mome raths outgrabe.

4 Pier Paolo Pasolini is famous all over the world as an art director. Actually, Pasolini is also a poet, a novelist and literary criticist. In this chapter I refer to a series of essays collected together in the book *Heretical Empiricism*. In my mind, such a title evokes one of the first works written by Gilles Deleuze: *Empiricism and Subjectivity*. Both are, as it were, works in progress, kinds of palimpsests of different essays composed in different times. It is clear enough, by the word "empiricism" in the two titles, that empiricism is the way where the subject passes throughout; not at all something stable and definitive.
5 The final part of Arthur Miller's *Death of a Salesman*, Requiem, when, at the end of the tragedy, Charley says:

> Nobody dast blame this man. You don't understand: Willy was a salesman. And for a salesman, there is no rock bottom to the life. He don't put a bolt to a nut, he don't tell you the law or give you medicine. He's a man way out there in the blue, riding on a smile and a shoeshine. And when they start not smiling back – that's an earthquake. And then you get yourself a couple of spots on your hat, and you're finished. Nobody dast blame this man. A salesman is got to dream, boy. It comes with the territory.

6 *Tarnation* is an extraordinary documentary filmed over 20 years of his life by Jonathan Caouette, a young American man. The movie is essentially about Jonathan's life and deals with Jonathan's schizophrenic mother and family. Caouette spent less than $300 on the budget and the movie received awards; it is an extraordinary example of a line of flight from Hollywood.

References

Aristotle (1997). *Poetics*. London: Penguin.
Artaud, A. (2004). *Oevres*. Paris: Gallimard.

Bachelard, G. (1992). *The Poetics of Reverie*. New York: Beacon.

Barbetta, P. (2015). Milan systemic family therapy. In J.L. Lebow et al. (eds), *Encyclopedia of Couple and Family Therapy*. Berlin: Springer.

Barbetta, P. (2016). *Locura y creacion*. Barcelona: Gedisa.

Barbetta, P. (2018). Percepts, affects and desire. In M. Nichterlein (ed.), *Putting the Deleuzian Machine to Work in Psychology. Annual Critical Psychology*. Issue 14, pp. 153–167. www.criticalinstitute.org/journals/arcp/9

Bateson, G. (1979). *Mind and Nature*. New York: Dutton.

Bateson, G. (2000a). Style, grace and information in primitive art. In *Steps to An Ecology of Mind*. Chicago, IL: The University of Chicago Press.

Bateson, G. (2000b). Double bind 1969. In *Steps to An Ecology of Mind*. Chicago, IL: The University of Chicago Press.

Bateson, G. (2000c). Form, substance and difference. In *Steps to An Ecology of Mind*. Chicago, IL: The University of Chicago Press.

Bateson, G. (2000d). Bali: The value system of a steady state. In *Steps to An Ecology of Mind*. Chicago, IL: The University of Chicago Press.

Bateson, G. (2000e). Pathologies of Epistemology. In *Steps to An Ecology of Mind*. Chicago, IL: The University of Chicago Press.

Bergson, H. (2012). *The Creative Mind: An Introduction to Metaphysics*. Mineola, NY: Dover Publications.

Boscolo, L. (1991). The systemic approach to the therapy of schizophrenia. In C. Eggers (ed.), *Schizophrenia and Youth*. Berlin, Heidelberg: Springer-Verlag.

Boscolo, L., Cecchin, G., Hoffman, L. and Penn, P. (1988). *Milan Systemic Family Therapy*. New York: Basic Books.

Carroll, L. (1941). *Through the Looking-Glass*. London: Macmillan.

Deleuze G. (1975/1976). *Lesson at Vincennes*. www.youtube.com/watch?v=tSCjYJ10I8c&t=2401s

Deleuze, G. (1986). *Cinema 1: The Movement-Image*. Minneapolis, MN: University of Minnesota Press.

Deleuze, G. (1989). *Cinema 2: The Time-Image*. Minneapolis, MN: University of Minnesota Press.

Deleuze, G. (1993a). *The Fold: Leibnitz and the Baroque*. New York: Continuum.

Deleuze, G. (1993b). *The Logic of Sense*. New York: Columbia University Press.

Deleuze, G. (1994). *Difference and Repetition*. New York: Columbia University Press.

Deleuze, G. (2008). *Two Regimes of Madness*. Los Angeles, CA: Semiotext(e).

Deleuze, G. (2018). *Foucault*. Padua: Orthotes.

Deleuze G. and Guattari, F. (1987). *A Thousand Plateaux: Capitalism and Schizophrenia*. Minneapolis, MN: University of Minnesota Press.

Deleuze G. and Guattari, F. (2013). *Anti-Oedipus, Capitalism and Schizophrenia*. London: Bloomsbury.

Foucault, M. (1964). *Madness and Civilization*. New York: Vintage.

Foucault, M. (2008). *Psychiatric Power (Lectures at the Collège de France)*. New York: Picador.

Foucault, M. (2011). *The Order of Things: An Archeology of Human Sciences*. New York: Random.

Guattari, F. (1995). *Chaosmosis: An Ethic-Aesthetic Paradigm*. Bloomington, IN: Indiana University Press.

Jakobson, R. (1986). *Hölderlin: L'arte della parola*. Genova: Il Melangolo.

Kermode, F. (2000). *The Sense of an Ending*. Oxford: Oxford University Press.

Lewin, A.L. (ed.) (1968). *Hippocrates Visits Democritus: Letters 10–12 of the Hippocratic Corpus*. Ithaca, NY: Cornell University Press.

Maturana, H. and Varela, F. (1980). *Autopoiesis and Cognition*. Boston, MA: Riedell.

Morin, E. (1990). *Science avec conscience*. Paris: Seuil.

Pasolini, P.P. (2005). *Heretical Empiricism*. New York: New Academia.

Piaget, J. (1973). *Introduction à l'épistemologié génétique: le pensée matématique*. Paris: PUF.

Richards, I.A. (1936). *The Philosophy of Rhetoric*. Oxford: Oxford University Press.

Schreber, P.D. (1988). *Memoires of My Nervous Illness*. New York: Book Review.

Steiner, G. (1989). *Real Presences: Is There Anything in What We Say?* Chicago, IL: The University of Chicago Press.

Stiegler, B. (2018). *The Neganthropocene*. London: Open Humanities Press.

Telfener, U. and Casadio, L. (2003). *Sistemica: voci e percorsi nella complessità*. Turin: Bollati.

von Foerster, H. (1982). *Observing Systems*. Seaside, CA: Intersystem Publications.

Chapter 3

Revolutionary Childhood

Maria Esther Cavagnis[1]

Introduction

The Order of Discourse for the Construction of Obedient Bodies

In therapeutic practices, there is a body of intertwining institutional meanings derived from the culture of which the therapist is part. Those categories define an agreed intelligibility, which makes visible some phenomena and others invisible. Thus, the persistence of beliefs and prejudices may appear in the guise of scientific gloss and actually reinforce subordination for adaptive and disciplinary purposes. Contemporary social debates have widely developed the effects of the dominant Occidental cultural models in matters of racial, sexual and gender inequalities, that colonization thus making visible the boundaries of those representations of the human (Burman, 2007, p. 7). This idea was developed by Foucault in his writings about the concept of Biopower to refer to the modern State practices which deploy different techniques in order to subdue bodies as a mechanism for controlling populations (Foucault, 2007).

The disciplinary societies that dominated the Occident from the seventeenth century to the end of the nineteenth organized and built establishments for confinement. The individual passes from one institution to another endlessly, each one with its own rules: first the family; immediately after, school; later the factory; and, if all those failed, the mental institution or prison, the institutions for confinement par excellence (Foucault, 1986). Children are educated inside the family, which becomes an abstract machine to produce obedient subjects, and this subjugation is codified and over codified in a phono-phallocentric culture[2] that worships the law as the foundation of society; reason above intuition and affections, and autonomy above the common.

Although Foucault and other authors in the social sciences, especially during recent decades, have tried to highlight the effects of this hetero-patriarchal culture on the normalization and naturalization of social inequalities, the effects of colonization on intergenerational relationships and models of childhood remain invisible. This is how the relationship adult–child

DOI: 10.4324/9780429437410-3

has come to be historically asymmetric and still remains unrevealed, underlying our therapeutic, educational and legal practices.

Traditional evolutionary psychology has become a normative frame that describes the child as an abstraction, without gender or social particularities. That abstraction does not only make inequalities invisible but reinforces them further as they become separate aspects of the body embedded in the material conditions of existence. "These models which do not consider the diversity of subjectivities, genders, races, geographies, class or social classes, educational levels, operate by pathologizing the differences" (Burman, 2013).

It makes me uneasy to hear parents, educators and therapists exclaiming at "a lack of limits" as an irrefutable diagnosis applied to any situation in which a child is seen as problematic. Similar judgments are made regarding other social problems: drug use, youth crime and other teenager criminal behaviors are all attributed to the failure of the family and/or school to discipline and control the "offenders". Permissiveness and adult loss of authority are blamed for social disruption and the deterioration of our way of life. Psychological theory follow along similar lines: the law of the father, hierarchical incongruity, etc. are clear examples of this position.

By the end of the nineteenth century there was a proliferation of studies that attempted to build models of "normal child development" producing a "child" subject from two points of view: first of all, the child "as not knowing" / not being, and second, the child as the object of an irrepressible urge for pleasure seeking that requires psy-control technologies for its restraint. I will refer to this further below. As a consequence of the assumption of the child's not knowing, mentioned above, childhood becomes *the* institution among the institutions: family-school-state. Children as "children" or "students" or "minors" according to the institution that "produces" them. The function of these institutions will be to model children's behavior and thinking: not only with regard to incest but also to relationships with parents, and others, with routines and with their own bodies.

The child is thus thought of as *becoming*, not yet *being*, one who, having been born helpless, must be led, tutored, to their final adult destiny in a movement between binary poles: from emotional to rational, dependent to independent, from fantasy to reality, from the empire of desire to the empire of the law. The child is the one who "does not yet think", whose witty remarks are childishly funny and amusing but never understood as thoughts. These practices give rise to a mechanism of interpretation which, unless the child echoes adult categories – what is "already known, and shared and expected" – their thoughts will be treated as deviant. Thus different disciplines come into being: child pedagogy, psychology, jurisprudence in relation to minors and the like. It is in this discourse domain that relations between adults and children in a culture are regulated, in the enduring presence of the greatest asymmetry in history. Eduardo Bustelo Grafigna expresses this idea in this way: the way we conceive of childhood, not the singular child's but that of all children collectively, gives rise to the new generation's views of the culture with respect to adults. Childhood is unquestionably situated in a relationship of dependence and subordination that leads to transformation into adulthood (Bustelo Graffigna, 2012).

The second characteristic of this "child subject" is that of an insatiable human being "by nature" who tends towards accumulation, destruction, tyranny of the other, and must therefore be disciplined as a form of social control. These arguments are so embedded in our language and practices and find such reinforcement through repetition that there is no room for problematization. Immature, incomplete, needy, unbearably natural... the child should be helped to understand the world and how best to adapt to its demands. The culture must restrain its destructive nature. From this perspective and for "the good of the child", what the responsible adult must do is to educate, train, subjectify, structure, into adulthood. The timeline goes back to the Ascetics as they sought for moral and spiritual perfection; the Calvinists declaring human absolute incapacity for good; the Puritans in their strict observance of norms of public and private moral conduct. And, of course, Christianity and the belief in original sin with the ensuing loss of grace.

At this point, I would like to address briefly the conceptualization of the Oedipus complex in the psychosexual development of the child, which, understood as universal structuring and social regulator, has been widely problematized by Deleuze and Guattari in *The Anti-Oedipus* (Deleuze and Guattari, 1980). They suggest that, in order to adequately fulfill the limiting functions of this destructive and egocentric nature, it is not only theories that have been developed, but also their respective technologies. The concepts of Ego, self, self-control, management, etc. are developments derived from them. This desired adaptation is achieved by an external control that will later become self-control derived from the development of a self that is able to internalize and govern it. That is to say, the theoretical model will determine the self (Foucault, 1990).

From Boundaries to Regulation: From Discipline to the Art of Living an Aesthetic Existence

In my opinion, what was revolutionary in Batesonian thought was his understanding of things in the contexts in which they occur, connecting different areas of knowledge that were thought to be separate. He brought the mind out of the brain "only to connect" it in terms of relationships. Those connections go through different worlds: animal, vegetable, human. The dichotomy is broken between the living and the non-living; nature and culture; the individual and the social; the interior and the exterior; the public and the private, establishing very different conceptual connections from those of the modernity present at the time.

What is the pattern that connects the crab to the lobster and the orchid to the primrose and all four of them to me? And me to you? And all the six of us to the amoeba in one direction and the backward schizophrenic in another?

(Bateson, 1982, p. 7)

As an ethnographer, in his investigations of the Iatmul people in New Guinea, Gregory Bateson studied a ritual called Naven. The Naven is destined to guarantee the passage to adulthood of a young man through practices of recognition and reaffirmation of the gender identity position and the relations between genders in the family and the community. The ethnographer described a pattern of relationship between men and women that works by successive cumulative and symmetrical interactions that we could describe as *the more of the one, the more of the other*. The rise continues until the climax is reached, which would be the result of a peak tension level in symmetrical communication, which needs resolution. This process is called schizogenesis (Bateson, 1990).

Significantly, the analysis of the Iatmul data led to the conceptualization of the "ethos" as the expression of a culturally standardized system of organization of the instincts and emotions of individuals. Bateson proposes that, over time, social rituals give rise to an "ethos": a dominant character, a system of habits. Those behaviors and sets of relationships are what the phenomenologist Alfred Schutz described as "taken for granted" or, to put it better, true ontologies.

A few years later, in an investigation developed in Bali with Margaret Mead, Bateson studied the system of raising and upbringing children in Balinese society, on the hypothesis that the character, or the base personality of the Balinese – what existential ontology defines as "normal" – depends on the system of raising and educating children: in "Balinese character", Bateson, says that no schismogenic sequences were observed in the relationship between adults (especially parents) and children in Bali (Bateson, 1985a).

The typical behavior of the Balinese child will be to initiate a cumulative interaction that grows into a tantrum. The mother will meanwhile play a spectator role. Bateson assumed that the repetition of this kind of interaction gradually led to the child's distrusting the intensity of relationships. The mother, by repressing her emotional involvement, showed that she felt uncomfortable with this type of interaction. The child, at the same time, learnt to regulate the excesses in the intensity of the relationship. In Western societies, this type of interaction would be described as an attachment deficit. However, this characteristic of Oriental societies will be the premise for human relations in which "a continuous plateau of intensity replaces the climax". This has been referred to as "oriental erotica" (Barbetta, 2018) (it should be noted that this is the text to which Deleuze refers when he refers to the origin of the title of one of the books he wrote with Guattari – *A*

Thousand Plateaus). These are very different ontologies, one based on the idea of "schismogenesis" – cumulative interaction – *escalation*, and the other based on the idea of a plateau, of continuous intensity – *regulation of intensities*. Given the tendency to the cumulative increase of tensions, a society can respond either by limiting the tensions when the boundary is reached or by continuously regulating that relationship to maintain it at the level of a metastable plateau. This has ontological consequences in the generation of an ethos, in which the pattern of regulation will produce a particular relational aesthetic, a way of being in a given culture. These are different processes of subjectivation that entail different political consequences, different social positions. A being with a tendency to destroy everything if we allow it needs the idea of an Ego that is able to control or limit the "voracious" one: an Ego that produces control effects. This is different from thinking in terms of regulation, in which we speak of a relationship, a pattern, that occurs "between" active agents. In the Batesonian terminology: "at least two descriptions are better than one" (Bateson, 1982, p. 122). It is a permanent regulatory process which does not end, a process of constant change and adjustment. The ethos, like any difference that makes a difference, is not fixed. Change and permanence, morphogenesis and morphostasis, are regulatory processes of life. Thus, the ontological effect of the Batesonian ethos is to erase dichotomies; the interior/exterior, individual/culture. How then does what the West calls interiority actually develop?

If I take into account the processes of incorporation and resistance present, I am unable to think of a passive child molded by the outside, who only internalizes object relations or patterns of relationship with adults in the coming into being of the self. I rather think of that child, the Batesonian child if you will, as participating actively in processes of multiple regulations with his environment. In this connection, let us explore the concept of *milieu*, which is not about the parents or the adults who take care of the child.

> Parents are themselves a milieu that children travel through: they go through its qualities and powers and make a map of them. It is not useful for us to think that children are limited by their parents before all else, and only through them gain access to milieus by extension or derivation. The father and mother are not the coordinates of everything. There is never a moment when children are not immersed in an actual physical and social milieu in which they are moving about, and in which the parents as persons simply play the roles of openers or closers of doors, guardians of thresholds, connectors or disconnectors of zones. The parents themselves always also occupy a position in a world that is not derived from them.
>
> (Deleuze, 1996)

Nor should milieu be understood as external, but rather in the immanent affinities that lead it to engage in specific associative relations since it is not related to "all" of the external world but only to a limited multiplicity of signs[2] (Nichterlein and Mors, 2017). Neither is it about total objects or their representation but rather about their partial qualities, intensities: those aspects capable of affecting it and being affected in turn (Uexküll, 1945). Referring to the Juanito[3] case Deleuze says:

> a milieu is made up of qualities, substances, powers, and events: the street, for example, with its materials (paving stones), its noises (the cries of merchants), its animals (horses) or its dramas (a horse slips, a horse falls down, a horse is beaten…).
>
> (Deleuze, 1996, p. 98)

The Dilemma of the Clinic: Docile or Revolutionary Bodies?

In relation to the clinic the question then is how to break away, how to find lines of flight from the systems that capture us. This was Foucault's concern in his later years, when he realized that the control of biopolitics is so intrusive that it has turned the idea of freedom more and more into an illusion (Foucault, 1999).

What is a revolutionary clinic about?

- It is not a matter of setting up a new regime of domination, much less of reinstating the one that was put in check by the symptomatic emergency, it is about making room for the creation of new possible worlds.
- It is about producing a change of regimes: breaking away from the regime of limitations to enable the regulation of relationships. Unlike limitations, regulations arise from within a relationship, not external universal patterns to judge what "ought to be" or is "good". It is a singular process with its own timing, modes and flows.
- It is a process between active, acting forces, between beings capable of mutual affectation, creating a way of living together both respecting difference and affirming itself in difference.
- It is not about the purpose of generating specific changes, it is about proposing a critical practice that helps to free life from stagnation and recover its vital natural flow.

The child resists capture. Many of the reasons for consultation are complaints from adults about this resistance: he/she does not obey, does not learn, does not communicate, etc. They assume that something "fails" in the child. The practice that I propose is far from control-driven, but rather aimed at listening to that voice and amplifying it, opening space so that what resists can unfold. I make use of two orientations: first, actual ongoing mapping rather than ready-made maps, and, second, paying close attention to small gestures that make sense beyond words to become signs of other possible gestures.

The Clinic as Cartographic Practice

In *A Thousand Plateaus* (Deleuze and Guattari, 2008), Félix Guattari and Gilles Deleuze proposed the principles of cartography and *tracing* to explain the concept of rhizome, linking these to the concepts of "assemblage", "machine" and "production of subjectivity". Cartography, map-making, is more of an action than a representation: rather than representing a world that is given, cartography involves the identification of new components, the creation of new relationships and territories, of new "machines". Cartography, map-making, contrasts with at least three classical traditions in the fields of production of knowledge: history, sociology and psychology. Guattari conceives cartography not simply as a technique of representation of given political subjectivities, but as an authentic revolutionary practice of aesthetic and political transformation.

In thinking about this topic Deleuze refers to Fernand Delingy (1913–1996), "weaver of networks, cartographer of wandering lines" (Deleuze, 1996, p. 99),[4] one of the greatest writers in the field of French social education, generally unknown in the Spanish and English speaking countries. Beginning in the 1950s, Deligny conducted a series of collectively run residential programs – he called them "attempts" (or *tentatives*, in French) – for children and adolescents with autism and other disabilities who would have otherwise spent their lives institutionalized in state-run psychiatric asylums. A member of the Tosquelles, with Guattari and Jean Ouri, he spent some time in "La Borde", a house Felix Guattari had bought in the middle of the Cévennes. He set up a clinic there for children diagnosed as autistic by Françoise Doltó and Maud Mannoni. His goal was to be close to this "singular ethnic group" as he called them, without too many preconceived ideas, with the aim of problematizing their diagnosis as seriously psychopathic, uneducable, and unrecoverable.

The children's everyday life was organized around connecting with nature, at their own pace, moved by their need to wander. This nomadic way of living is related to that of archaic ethnic groups, especially in terms of the paths the children followed in their daily itineraries, in the style of those tribes that wander along uncharted paths, free displacements. "They sought to develop "a practice that would exclude from the outset interpretations referring to some code" – anticipating, by several decades, some of the central tenets of the neurodiversity and autistic self-advocacy movements: "We did not take the children's ways of being as scrambled, coded messages addressed to us" (Deligny, 2015).

How to Historicize without Annulling the Becomings?

Psychological theories often involve historicizing practices more closely related to archeology than to cartography in the way of shifting plates containing memorials, commemorative, monumental conceptions of the past that live on in memory. The search is rather a probe into the depths of layer upon layer of the tectonic plates of memory of experience.

The point is not to ignore history, but rather to problematize the ways of historicizing the past. Just as history is impossible, it is not possible to live without history. Whenever there has been humanity there was history. Yet, how far can we trust history when we know it fails to include difference? The problem is to try to make a carbon copy, a copy that represents the past, as accurately as possible, unique, in the sense of a single one, not singular. As Deleuze and Guattari say in *The Anti-Oedipus,* the problem is linearity in the relationship between history and becoming – subordinating becoming to history, the return to a personal history that refers to "father", "mother": the search for a particular origin, the buried objects, found along the trodden paths of memory or even oblivion (Deleuze and Guattari, 1980).

Unlike the copy, a *tracing* enables transfer in such a way that each map can show difference from the next: a record of errancy, of the displacements between one map and the other. Like Deligny's tracings, each one of them describes the singular trajectory of a day for each one of the children with whom he lived and, by transferring each of them on paper, he created a map with all its variations, closures, exits, multiplicities and regularities. A map which to be read without annulling its forces requires going from bottom to top, following its singular displacements.

> There is not only a reversal of directions, but also a difference in nature: the unconscious no longer deals with persons and objects, but with trajectories and becomings; it is no longer an unconscious of commemoration but one of mobilization, an unconscious whose objects take flight rather than remain buried in the ground.
>
> (Deleuze, 1996, p. 102)

Affects and Intensities

In our practice, we are compelled to follow the children's trajectories, to make maps of their movements as well as their affections and intensities. The maps that can be drawn are not only of extension, of spatial trajectories, we can also draw maps of intensity, which express the affective constellations that sustain the movement. The two maps, that of trajectories and that of affections, refer one to the other (Deleuze, 1996). It is not only a matter of attending to their movements, their thematic paths, the sequences of their games or their verbalizations, but also of paying special attention to the affectations present on those pathways. Something of a different order that moves us, a restlessness, a speed, a different intensity. It may only last an instant so it is imperative to be very attentive.

The Clinic of Small Gestures

It is necessary to undo that face so as to become. Becoming is change in the way we relate to the familiar elements of our existence. An encounter is necessary for new sense to arise, *we* only become in relation to something else as we make contact with the outside, with those signs we encounter and which bring us out of ourselves, force us to respond in a different way: a *gesture* that escapes control of the face showing difference in repetition, creating a new other, as in art, an act also of political resistance.

In the collaborative making of the film *Le Moindre Geste*, based on his observation of autistic ways of living, Fernand Deligny re-creates a world that is no longer ruled by language (*Le Moindre Geste*, 2007). A world in which words, perhaps, no longer *belong* to anyone. They are abandoned; left there contextless, just there. Don't try to understand! ... Stop looking! Attention is focused on the gesture, on the ephemeral, on the microscopic, in the chaos of the incomprehensible, of what is and what is not, not only what happens, but what *is* happening, the tiniest thing... A gesture, a minimal gesture. An event that bursts in and becomes experience (Deligny, 2013).

Gesture is flesh, rather than word, and its power lies in its potential to shatter meaning or at least make cracks in it as a given, thus changing the real. Meaning is imprisonment, unwitting gesture is a revolutionary sign, a new sense, and looks to the future. And, for its potential for transformation in an encounter with the other to be retained, it should remain uninterpreted, unexplained. In the clinic, it is usually the child, whose gesture escapes the "hard face" of dominant discourse, who forces us to think against given representation. It is the difference that makes a difference, and that is what we can truly call *thinking*. Gesture is a sign that has the power to elude given representation. There is thought when the active forces act, and the world of representation is transformed anew. Thinking is seeing and speaking only if the eye looks on "visibilities" rather than on things; only if language goes beyond words and phrases reaching out for new meaning.

The Session: The Possibility of the Event

The family session can give us the opportunity to map instead of simply record. It has the potential to let the new arise or it may just become obliteration of difference. It is a space in which to problematize, raise questions about what the child can do, and their resistances, their captures and their powers; a space where to ask ourselves what are the processes of subjectification at work and what the possibilities for the child to find new ways of folding, of putting together a self, an aesthetic existence with the greatest possible margins of freedom.

Talking with the child, not "talking about the child" (Glasserman, 1980).

The family session is an opportunity to talk *with* the child, not *about* the child. This cannot simply mean putting meanings into words. In general, talk is what is mostly restricted in the child's language acquisition process and they tend to find fuller expression in drawing or play. In our adult culture, however, what does not translate into words does not exist. The predominance of the signifier over the sign is the preferred mode of expression, particularly in psy-culture. If we respect children's modes of expression, they will participate actively in the session. In our own practice,[5] we do not keep a traditional, confidential clinical history of the parents' stories of their child's development and their concerns. The child is always present and actively participating in interactions from the first meeting and is brought in to express himself in whatever way he or she chooses.

Talking with the child is linked to "thinking with him/her". To quote Foucault: "Thinking is between what can be seen and what can be said" (Ball, 2001). To think with a child is to recognize their position as equals in the relationship and to prevent the arbitrary authority of the dominant discourse from submitting them to it. Thinking is also power, that is, weaving relations of forces. Barbetta (2004) brings up the Bakhtinian concept of "heteroglossia" in the clinic to refer to the coexistence of multiple languages – *idiolects* – in relational terms such as exemplified in a family session. Some of these languages are dominant, others more or less subsumed, but all of them present there, with the possibility of becoming *an-other* in the flow of those multiple languages. Sometimes one of the subsumed languages emerges at a particular moment, in a singular way in the space between what can be seen and what can be said (Barbetta, 2004).

"These children have some strange ideas, notions". There is a popular saying in Argentina: "Beware of children: they will talk!" And it is true, they are well-founded fears. Children will speak their minds, express themselves, they are born practitioners of parrhesia. Foucault's last consideration is to refer to the risky cynical practice of parrhesia as the shaper of life (Foucault, 2017). This is why they must be "civilized", domesticated. And yet, unless there is a very subtle balance, the outcome might be subjugation.

There are also those who will stand as spokesperson for the child in the role of interpreters: "I understand what he meant", thus hegemonizing a univocal reading: "because I am the mother" or "because I have known him longer", or "because I am his therapist", or whatever. Another way of crushing the singularity of the expression is from the rigorous standards of universal theoretical readings either in terms of unconscious conflict, educational failure or references to conventional developmental stages.

The attributions of influence are numberless: blame it on television, school, the mother or the grandmother or any other "outsiders", who assume the child as unable to think for himself/herself, just imitates, etc. These influences invoke a sense of alienation, which contributes to the delegitimization of the child's thinking. A dramatic example of this is false parental alienation syndrome, in which the value of a child's word is annulled, attributing it to the influence of one of the parents against the other in cases of destructive divorce.

Drawing in Session: The Event Is Not What Happens, It Is Within What Happens

We practice as a team of child therapists, some of whom are experienced, others in training. Our rooms are furnished with blackboards, which allow the child, if he or she chooses, to draw during the session, the drawings being there for everyone to see, rather than concealed by the privacy of the sheet. While the session takes place and the adults talk about the child or what they feel about the child, the children choose how to participate, talking at times, and at other times maybe just drawing. They are all wrapped up in their work with all the earnestness involved in the game. Behind the camera, the way these different languages come into being is particularly clear. As if on a screen, the blackboard is filled with lines, images added, erased, superimposed one way or another. The conversation of the adults takes place in "audio mode", with almost no movement except for some minimal gestures, to which we must be very attentive. Children actively participate in the experience in "image-in-motion mode" almost like on the cinema screen where the audio and the image do not necessarily coincide, but rather refer to each other. The child does not graphically represent what is spoken, but neither is their casual drawing detached from what happens there. This brings to mind the warp and weft of a fabric. The figures turn into a field of intensities and affectations. The order, the organization of the spoken discourse and the image together create a composition that is far removed from a simple "illustration"; the composition creates a new image. The challenge is to listen well to that parallel language in its capacity of affectation, which, if ignored would vanish altogether. To make room for it without interpreting with the hegemony of a single given signifier or a symbol of something else, but as a pure expression of the child's process of subjectivation. And when they find that place or position, children usually allow us to enter their world and we may wander with them following their maps of pathways and affections.

Children's Graphic Production Reading Criteria

Until now the criteria for reading children's graphics have been limited to assumptions of meanings, unconscious-referred meanings, ostensibly supported by analogies (read "the father" for "the Sun", "the mother" for "the smaller figure"). The child's drawings and the accompanying verbalizations have been interpreted in such a way that rhythm, melody, dance are neutralized, minimizing their plasticity, the actual chromatic range of what is usually missed in pictograms. A drawing should be read in the same way as we listen to or read a story, or watch a movie. Therapists often find children's drawings unintelligible unless they are accompanied by verbalization. However, there is nothing like child art to study the repetition of difference as a difference, avoiding any attempt to reduce it to mere representation. Drawing, like music, is in a privileged position, free from analogies, for us to attend to its form, which is untranslatable. Children's drawings have been over-interpreted and we have convinced young therapists in training that the essential thing is to think about the content of an interpretation (of what is spoken) rather than help them to develop their awareness of what can potentially affect them.

In our clinic when the child draws in a session we do not think of the drawing as an expression of an unconscious or intrapsychic conflict; we rather see ourselves in the role of participants in what is happening, what is affecting that body, what forces the session is bringing into play, affecting what is happening there and then and at the same time affected by it. It is about composing each time, generating a singular encounter that does not respond to any previous nosography or conception of deep structures.

Hernán, an Argentinian boy of nine years old, was under medication for a school phobia crisis. In the latest episode he suddenly ran away from school and crossed the street ignoring the lights. He ran home, about five or six blocks from school and when he got there, he was apparently calm. The psychiatrist, who made the diagnosis, had suggested an overinvolved bond with his mother, which at his age should have already been overcome by relational psychotherapy standards. Later, in a session which Maria Esther was supervising, Hernán drew a huge head, with a transparent brain. With intricate patterns inside and a huge red stain on its throat resembling blood. The therapists and the parents started to talk with great concern for Hernán's older brother who is addicted to drugs and frequently steals to buy them. Hernán's mother had seemingly previously been unaware of this situation. During this conversation Hernán, for the first time, was able to express his fear of leaving the house because he felt that this would put his brother at risk of going out to steal and buy drugs and possibly being killed by the police. In this way a symptom occurred in a fold from the outside going beyond what was strictly familiar. A process of subjectivation took place in which extra-familial forces broke into the familiar and questioned it and it all became so threatening that Hernán became the caretaker of his older brother. Systemic psychotherapists are perhaps used to thinking this way about school refusal as a symbol of something else. However, we are suggesting that it is important to pay attention not just to the familiar relationship in this case between Hernán and his parents or brother, but also to the shape and intensity of other forces, in this case the huge head, the transparent brain and the blood red stain, telling us something about the perceived danger and brutality of the police.

Semiotics, Sign: Maybe It Is Not About Objects, But Rather About Affections, Intensities

Drawings, gestures, wanderings in space, at play or in conversation, they are expressions that seek a way out. To interpret is to cancel, to suffocate singularity. The semiotics of gesture, mimicry, play, configure an intensive line that works on its own, and is often more free with children: *tracing* rather than representation. The difference is considerable. In the tracing there is not a shred of representation. That work of art is nothing less than a gesture. While they are wrapped up in their drawing in the same way that they are entangled in language an event takes place that upsets the balance of local power. Deligny, connecting tracing with music, says that those two or rather multiple languages build a composition, create a chord. "'Accord', a word that etymologically may refer to either or both, the heart and/or the string, it is not consent or compliance, but rather dis-cord from which different frequency relationships will resonate" (Deligny, 2013, p. 151).

Bateson Art, Grace and Style

The drawing, as well as other non-linguistic objects, has the capacity to evade any form of colonialism. An image can become an event capable of upsetting the balance of local power and give rise to moments of "grace" in the Batesonian sense, since they can produce new affectations. Bateson, referring to primitive art, proposes man as a being who has fallen from "grace", a state which animals, as well as God (and children I would add), still enjoy. He affirms that art is a way of searching for that lost grace and maintains that grace is fundamentally a matter of integration. What is to be integrated are the diverse aspects of mind, especially those multiple levels, one end of which is called "conscious" and the other "unconscious". To achieve grace, the reasons of the heart have to be integrated with the reasons of reason (Bateson, 1985b): how is this integration contained or codified in the work of art and particularly in children's art? The reasons of the heart, or of the unconscious, are coded and patterned in totally different ways from the rules of language. And, since much of conscious thought is structured in terms of the logic of language, the logic of the unconscious is doubly inaccessible. It is not only that the conscious mind finds access to that material difficult, but also that when that access is achieved, in dreams, art, poetry, religion, intoxication and other similar states, the insurmountable problem of translation remains.

Following Bateson we can say that "every picture tells a story", and this generalization applies to most of art, but it is not about reducing everything to the analysis of history. That aspect of the work of art that can be more easily put into words – the mythology related to the subject – is what I do not want to analyze. The objective is not instrumental. It's not about overriding the transformation by "decoding the message". This would be just a neat way of stealing the body or denying the problem.

"*Le style est l'homme même*" **(The style is the man himself).**[6]

Graphic production, beyond what is represented, has a code / its own style, its stroke, its expressive intensities, its rhythm, its planes, its composition. It becomes pure line, pure color. What is implicit in style? The code by which the perceived is transformed into line, color or plane is a source of information about the child's experience, an expression of their affectations. What matters is the transformation rules themselves, not so much the message but the code. We need a conceptual framework that enables us to see graphic expression, like other creative productions, as something internally endowed with a singular pattern and at the same time as a folding of a larger universe, with its own patterns, like the culture and the institutions to which it gives rise either in a general or singular way. The family, the child's family; the school, the child's school; the mother / father-mother / father etc.

Young children want to play/draw, they do not have a fixed plan about what games to play / what to draw. It depends on what they can find and the path is accidental. It will not do to under interpret, to postulate that in these wanderings each object found or created or each drawing made symbolizes the inevitable "mum and dad". The code of children's production, like that of any art object, is iconic, unlike verbal language, which is arbitrary and digitally coded.

In Opening Mode

Before a system that aims to block desire, circumscribe it to segmental lines, which aims to make each individual appear "modulated" by the same frequency, what must be done is to seek *lines of flight* emerging or that can be traced, where the unexpected can make an appearance: the event, the "revolutionary becoming" that produces a transformation". This is how art takes segments of the real and deterritorializes them to turn them into partial enunciators of what cannot be said. The clinic should help to unlock the creative potential of expression and enunciation that has been silenced. Let the "occurrence", the "nonsense", the "madness" happen so that new networks may arise as a form of resistance. The function of the network is to resist and create.

In childhood are to be found the forces that transform the status quo; it carries the new, the potency of the newly created, and therefore becomes a substantive time of social change. It is no longer thought of, as in the view of socialization, as something to be cast in the adult mold, but rather represents the possibility of a change for the better. In short, it is about freeing life from stagnation. An encounter will become therapeutic only if it is capable of releasing creative power, a new force: The revolutionary becoming of the therapeutic process does not obey conscious purpose; it is rather to be found in the potency of the event.

Notes

1 I am a director and coordinator of the team specialized in clinical assistance to families with children, carrying out training and supervision of graduate students.
2 Derrida, Jacques (1930–2004) in *Plato's Pharmacy*, coined the term, today used in linguistics and sociology for the use of one term, man, as a generalization for the other(s) woman, people. The term man excludes women and indicates a male bias (Derrida, 1975).

3 *Umwelt*, in German, a powerful concept created by Jacob von Uexkull, an anti-Darwinian biologist, to refer to the "subjective experience of the animal". *Milieu*, in French, refers to an imminent, not transcendent, view of the environment. We do not relate to a medium that is out there already given and equal for all the organisms that live there. It occurs in relationships with some specific aspects of everything available as virtual or potential.

4 Little Hans was a five-year-old boy with a phobia of horses. Freud wrote a summary of his treatment of Little Hans, in 1909, in a paper entitled "Analysis of a phobia in a five-year-old boy". Freud attempted to demonstrate that the boy's fear of horses was related to his Oedipus complex and the castration-threat anxiety caused by this conflict.

5 Wander... a word that Deligny often uses in relationship to mapping the wander lines: *vaguer*, a verb that shares a root with the French noun for "wave" (Burk and Porter alternate between translating this word as "wandering" and "drifting"). Like the French word *vague*, drift carries with it a sense of the movement of water, as in drifting down a river (a figuration that also recalls Deligny's comparison of his group's provisional encampments to rafts afloat on a sea of language). Indeed, Deligny's language continuously evokes a kind of bodily letting go – an attenuation of subjective agency and conscious intentionality, as when one surrenders to a powerful ocean current. This quality is central to what Deligny is trying to evoke with the *lignes d'erre*, which seem to register an epistemological slackening of the distinction between the human subject and the non-human forces it encounters in a given environment.

6 FYP (The Family and Couple Foundation), an institution founded in 1979 by Maria Rosa Glasserman and Adolfo Loketek, are pioneers in the training of systemic family therapists in Latin America.

7 Leclerc de Buffon, G.L. (1707–1788), French naturalist, a member of the French Academy, his inaugural address being the celebrated "Discourse sur le style", 1753.

References

Ball, S. (2001). *Foucault y la educacion*. Buenos Aires: Paideia.

Barbetta, P. (2004). El juego de las disidencias en las narrativas terapéuticas: del monologo a la heteroglosia. *Sistemas familiares y otros sistemas humanos*, 20(1), 22–36.

Barbetta, P. (2018). *La terapia familiare sistemica nel tempo della complessità*. www.aiems.eu/18_numero

Bateson, G. (1982). *Espiritu y naturaleza*. Buenos Aires: Amorrortu.

Bateson, G. (1985a). Estilo, gracias e información en el arte primitivo. In *Pasos hacia una ecologia de la mente*. Buenos Aires: Lohlé.

Bateson, G. (1985b). El caracter balinés. In *Pasos hacia una ecologia de la mente*. Buenos Aires: Lohlé.

Bateson, G. (1990). *Naven*. Buenos Aires: Jucar.

Burman, E. (2007). Introduction. In *Deconstructing Developmental Psychology*. Abingdon: Routledge.

Burman, E. (2013). Desiring development? Psychoanalytic contributions to anti-developmental psychology. *International Journal of Qualitative Studies in Education*, 26(1), 56–74.

Bustelo Graffigna, E. (2012). Notas sobre infancia y teoria: un enfoque latinoamericano. *Salud Colectiva*, 8(3), 287–298.

Deleuze, G. (1996). Lo que dicen los niños. In *Crítica y clínica*. Barcelona: Anagrama.

Deleuze, G. and Guattari, F. (1980). El antiedipo. In *Capitalismo y esquizofrenia*. Buenos Aires: Paidos.

Deleuze, G. and Guattari, F. (2008). Mil mesetas. In *Capitalismo y esquizofrenia*. Valencia: Pre-Textos.

Deligny, F. (2013). *Lo arácnido y otros textos*. Buenos Aires: Cactus.

Deligny, F. (2015). *Los vagabundos eficaces*. Buenos Aires: Universitat Oberta de Catalunya.

Derrida, J. (1975). La farmacia de Platón. In *La diseminacion*. Madrid: Fundamentos.

Foucault, M. (1986). *Vigilar y castigar*. Madrid: Siglo XXI Editores.

Foucault, M. (1990). *Tecnologias del yo*. Barcelona: Paidos.

Foucault, M. (1999). *La ética del cuidado de sí como practica de la libertad*. Barcelona: Paidós.

Foucault, M. (2007). *Nacimiento de la bio-política*. Buenos Aires: Fondo de Cultura Economica.

Foucault, M. (2017). *La parrêsía*. Madrid: Biblioteca Nueva, S.L.

Glasserman, M. (1980). *La práctica de la terapia familiar*. Buenos Aires: Psicolibro.

Le Moindre Geste. (2007). [Film] Directed by J.P. Deligny, F. Daniels. SLON.

Nichterlein, M. and Mors, J. (2017). *Deleuze and the Psychology*. Abingdon and New York: Routledge.

Uexküll, J.V. (1945). *Ideas para una concepción biológica del mundo*. Buenos Aires: Espasa'Calpe.

Chapter 4

Thoughts from the Outside[1]

Inga-Britt Krause

Introduction

Deleuze and Guattari rarely speak about culture in the abstract. Yet much of their work is influenced by anthropologists and anthropological material (Bialecki, 2018). In *Anti-Oedipus* (2004) there are references to Lévi-Strauss, Leach, Malinowki and Turner, and examples from societies in which orientations to life, relationships, politics and economics are quite foreign to Westerners. Examples are found in references to the Dogon (Griaule, 1965), the Ndembu (Turner, 2000) and the Tiv (Bohannan and Bohannan, 1953) in discussions of kinship, ritual and economic exchange. Amongst other things they argue that "oedipalization" as a form of "solution on the scale of the individual and the restricted family" (Deleuze and Guattari, 2004 , p. 185), by which I think they mean the nuclear family, is an example of intimate colonial education. They write: "Culturalists and ethnologists have demonstrated that institutions are primary in relation to affects and structures. For structures are not mental, they are present in things (*elles sont dans les choses*), in the form of social production and reproduction" (Deleuze and Guattari, 2004, , p. 189, emphasis in original). The starting point is thus not universals, because universals "explain nothing and must themselves be explained" (Deleuze and Guattari, 1991, p. 7), nor is it concepts because "you will know nothing through concepts unless you have first created them" (Deleuze and Guattari, 1991, p. 7). However, concepts easily slide into being considered universals in any discipline and in this hidden way represent particular worldviews, even if we do not notice this. Through their critique Deleuze and Guattari aim to provide an altogether different starting point than standard Western philosophy or Western social science, one which endeavors to be inclusive and avoids doing everything as we always have done it and then adding a bit of "culture" or "race" or "institutionalized difference" at the end. Although the critique in *Anti-Oedipus* apparently is leveled at psychoanalysis this book and a subsequent one, *A Thousand Plateaus* (Deleuze and Guattari, 2013), aim wider to include capitalism as a mode of production and reproduction and therefore the concepts and frameworks of

DOI: 10.4324/9780429437410-4

all of us who exist and work within this type of society and economy. Accordingly, systemic psychotherapy and systemic psychotherapists also have these problems. That there was a problem in the developing discipline of systemic psychotherapy was demonstrated with the near fatal split (at least for some years and between certain persons) between Bateson and his colleagues in Palo Alto around the publication of *Pragmatics of Human Communication* (Watzlawick et al., 1967) when Bateson felt that the team had left "culture" out (Harries-Jones, 1995; Krause, 2007, 2012). The extent of this problem has been becoming evident in the last decade or so and my turning to the inspiration of Deleuze and Guattari now is an attempt to overcome, or at least to address, this problem, and because of the influence of Bateson to go back to a time before the split to seek a new direction, which although we may not have taken it, is nevertheless present in the discipline, its history and in the possibilities it offers now.

The problem is this: How to understand someone else? Or how to understand another system/context? The ideas of Deleuze and Guattari suggest that in most disciplines this involves some reliance on the Oedipus complex as a starting point and with it a view of the family in which desire is considered a lack, and which beginning with the child is extended to the adult, to the family, and then to the social organization and in our case to capitalist consumerism. This is the way desire can be fulfilled for families mostly separated from economic production and in which, in turn, relationships are symbolized by the oedipal relationship.[2] The standard systemic emphasis on context therefore does not necessarily ensure a way out of this cycle of reproduction, unless we rethink the "context" and the dynamics in it. A self-fulfilling process is in motion, and we may not notice our contribution to it.

However, contexts offer many possibilities, possibilities which may point to new lines of development or lines of flight (Guattari, 2016). In this chapter I turn my attention to a particular local context in order to examine the possibilities, which may enhance my understanding of a particular piece of work and particular events, which took place in therapy. In focusing on events I follow Deleuze's understanding of radical empiricism which

> does not present a flux of the lived that is immanent to a subject and individualised in that which belongs to itself. *It presents only events, that is possible worlds as concepts, and other people as expressions of possible worlds and conceptual personae.*
>
> (Deleuze and Guattari, 1991, pp. 47–48; my emphasis)

The emphasis on events is a bit like the emphasis on process, but I consider it more punctuated and more overdetermined because of the significance of events and what they may articulate and what is not obvious on the surface. It is precisely in the interpretation of events that we educate, and in that process we are in danger of colonizing.

I am interested in what we may understand is behind particular events and the possibilities they may offer. For myself as a therapist I am interested in how I understand a particular event and my involvement in it. Although I am immensely inspired by the writings of Deleuze and Guattari I am not a captive of their ideas. I have also been inspired by the writings of several social anthropologists as will become clear. I turn first to describing the central event, which has attracted my attention in a piece of therapeutic work and I shall give more information about the context of the event and my work with one particular family. I then place the event into a theoretical framework, some aspects of which are familiar to systemic psychotherapists, others perhaps more familiar to social anthropologists. In what follows I address the question I posed above, namely how do we understand someone else or another context? This will be followed by a discussion referring to ideas, which I find useful in trying to capture an understanding of the event. It is here I refer to Deleuze and Guattari as well as to other thinkers known to systemic psychotherapists such as Maturana and to social anthropologists such as Strathern (2004), Ingold (2017) and Viveiros de Castro (2017). The inspiration from Bateson is never far from the ideas which these writers express. Here, then, I introduce ideas about kinship and families from social anthropology to the systemic field. These may seem complex at first but I attempt to show how such interdisciplinary thinking, which emphasizes the dynamic of families and family systems as well as the multiplicity of positions such systems afford, can enrich thinking and practice in this field.

The Five, Nay Six Women and Girls in Different Shades of Aliveness

There are six women (including myself) in this account. There are men too, but they are much more shadowy and I have never met them. There are daughters, sisters, mothers, grandmothers and granddaughters, and these positions are occupied at different times by different persons, who therefore at different times stand in a different relationship to each other. For example, a mother is also a daughter, a granddaughter is also a sister, a grandmother is also a daughter etc. Although the men and boys are absent, they are not insignificant. There are sons, fathers, lovers and brothers, but what takes place happens separate from their direct involvement in the events in the therapy room, although they may be instrumental in the way events are presented and how they do and do not unfold. The work is taking place now (at the time of writing) in the UK and so the family has lived through post-WWII capitalism and now lives within late capitalism, and even if the family relationships do not conform to ideal expectations of "family" in this context, they are as shaped and influenced by the "family spirit" (Bourdieu, 1998, pp. 64–74) of capitalism, as I am myself. This causes difficulties. For example, housing is built for conventional nuclear families, but in this family none of the adult children have separated and definitively left home and this in itself has practical and financial implications. The family is mostly white, partly of Irish, partly of English London working class descent. Those who have been employed have worked as laborers and in domestic services such as cleaning and clothes washing. At the moment only one person, a man, is in employment.

The event upon which I want to focus took place during the spring of 2018. I had been working with the family for several years and had become familiar with the tensions and pulls and pushes, blind allies and stuckness, which they all had experienced, but which had been communicated to me in different ways by the three persons who attend the therapy, the daughter/granddaughter of 14, Olivia, the mother/daughter of 30, Sarah, and the grandmother/mother of 58, Margaret. Occasionally, I also met with Maja (four), Olivia's younger sister from a different father and daughter of Sarah. I have known that Chloe, an aunt, sister and daughter, one year older than Sarah, had died at the age of 14, 16 years or so ago. There have been other deaths in the family to which I will return. The session upon which I want to focus began with talk about the ways in which Sarah and Chloe were alike and then turned to the way Chloe died. Both Sarah and Chloe had contracted meningitis, Sarah after Chloe. Chloe had died in hospital and although Sarah was seriously ill in hospital too, she was not in such a serious condition as Chloe and survived. Margaret had been in an impossible situation and had not been able to be with Sarah and care for her as she had been at Chloe's bedside. Following these tragic events, Sarah was and to some extent still is in a crisis. She was diagnosed with depression, put herself in repeated danger in the streets, became pregnant at 15 and gave birth to Olivia. Sarah was repeatedly abused by Olivia's father and Margaret became Olivia's official carer when Olivia was three years old. Margaret herself had a breakdown after Chloe's death. She described how she had been in bed for weeks focusing on the lampshade all day waiting for her sleeping medication so that she could escape into sleep from her thoughts. Sarah's breakdown after her sister's death is described by her as feeling the loss and feeling uncared for by her mother. She finds it difficult to talk about Chloe even now.

Margaret spoke about all of this in a session after Chloe's then boyfriend had called her on the anniversary of Chloe's death (as he regularly does) and told her about all the things he had accomplished since they last spoke, and Margaret said that she realized that in her family things are just the same, that nothing has happened and that they are stuck. Margaret then told me that Chloe's ashes are still in a plastic bag in the airing cupboard in her house. She had tried to bury them, but had not succeeded in making the necessary arrangements and Sarah and her two brothers had also stopped her. It has taken one brother several years before he has been able to mention Chloe's name and even now will not easily speak of her. Sarah will not allow her mother to move the ashes and Margaret said that she was very reluctant to open up the subject for discussion. At the end of the session I said that I thought that Chloe was sitting there in the cupboard presiding over the stuckness and I wondered how she could come alive again in a different way.

In a subsequent session with Sarah and Margaret (Olivia was seen by a child psychotherapist and at that time did not join our sessions) we again returned to the stuckness, which was also referred to by Sarah. I mentioned the stuckness and Margaret said that if I was referring to Chloe's ashes, she did not agree with me. She said that she had asked other people who have lost a child and they also keep their child's ashes in the house, so the stuckness has nothing to do with Chloe's death. She agreed that they are stuck but that this had to do with all the other deaths in the family. Sarah had tears in her eyes and said that she does not want to talk about Chloe, and the conversation moved on to how Olivia is afraid of her own death, but according to Margaret not concerned about the death of others. Sarah said that Maja has asked about the death of Chloe but also about the death of her father, Maja's grandfather, worrying about whether she, her mother, will die. Sarah said that she replied that she does not know when she will die because she does not want to reassure Maja about something she does not know. The theme of the stuckness returned and Sarah and Margaret said that they would like that to change. Sarah summarized a situation which she would have liked to have been different: when Maja performed in her nativity play at school, Margaret, Maja's grandmother, Sarah's mother, had rushed up and given Maja a hug, while Sarah had felt left behind wanting to shout: "Hello, I am here, I am her mother".

Family Doubles and Partial Connections

Bateson described schismogenesis in his study of Iatmul society (Bateson, 1958) and particularly in relation to the Naven ceremony in which certain familial relationships were ritually enacted. Since then schismogenesis is, if referred to at all in systemic psychotherapy, explained as a generic theory of relationships pointing to the way in which a relationship may be reproduced by its own dynamic. This used to be explained to students using the examples of nagging wives and avoidant husbands (complementary) or two parties in an escalating argument (symmetrical) (Watzlawick et al., 1967). Why these particular behaviors or emotions were considered to be fitting examples has not, to my knowledge at least, been explained and I doubt that many students or trainees have asked. What was therefore lost to systemic psychotherapists, but which was central in Bateson's analysis of the Naven ritual, was why persons behave like this in certain contexts. The particular became accepted as the general (universal) and therefore the connections between emotional outlooks and wider social and economic structures and processes were lost. Systemic psychotherapists were left with a general theory more or less matched to the political and economic contexts in which systemic psychotherapy tends to operate without an acknowledgement of this circularity. The particular expression/behaviors of schismogenesis could either be seen as a natural (universal) state of affairs or as pathological subjectivity. This is central to the problem as outlined above.

In schismogenesis there is already a relationship between the two parties or sides before they go into the dynamic of the process. In the case of the Naven ritual the participants already stand in a relation of mother's brother and sister's son to each other, and this has wider connotations with respect to the arrangement and position of descent groups and other lines of descent and filiation[3] in Iatmul society (Bateson, 1958; Krause, 2007). One could say that these wider relationships, which are political and economic as well as emotional and familial, are expressed through the individual and subjective relationships between persons who stand in a relation of mother's brother/sister's son to each other. The mother's brother, the *wau* denotes certain ideas, feelings and outlooks to Iatmul people as does the sister's son, the *laua*. The two kinship terms denote ideas, feelings and behaviors, which already are there in the expectations of Iatmul people. In addition, if we stop focusing on the narrowness of the nuclear family, we also see that a mother's brother is at least potentially also a sister's son and vice versa, sister's sons are potentially also mother's brothers. There is then something of the mother's brother in the sister's son and this will be so, even if to varying extents, in every relationship. There will always be a social dimension in a relationship, which is there before any relationship between particular persons (Deleuze and Guattari, 2004, , p. 170).

This is also the case in the family of Olivia, Sarah and Margaret. The dynamic between them circles around the relationships of sisters, mothers and daughters. Olivia is a daughter to Sarah, but at times she is also her sister especially when the relationship is considered from the point of view of Margaret, her grandmother, who is her carer, a position she holds via Sarah, who sometimes feels displaced. Olivia is of course also potentially a mother, something everyone views with fear as Olivia is coming near to the age Sarah was when she gave birth to her. Olivia is also a sister to Maja, a relationship they hold via Sarah and which is imbued with their own as well as Sarah's ambivalences about sisterhood. Sarah is a daughter to Margaret, a sister to her dead sister Chloe, and a mother to Olivia and Maja, and Margaret is a mother (grandmother), a daughter to her own mother who passed away a couple of years ago and a sister to her brother. As I have hinted, these different kinship positions and the possibilities they afford become further multistranded as a result of the particular circumstances of this family. This, I think, is what came to the fore in the session I have outlined above, when Margaret acted in her role of main carer and Sarah felt she had to remind her that *she* is the mother, echoing, it seems to me, that Sarah felt that she was not so much of a daughter as her beloved sister and not so much of a mother as her own mother. While you would expect ambivalences about kinship relationships in all families, in this family the tensions between love or care and ambivalence frequently stand in the way of a freer, lighter, more hopeful outlook. I have myself felt caught up in this as I too am a mother, a daughter and a sister-in-law and I, too, was brought up by my maternal grandmother. I recognized/felt in my own body, as it were, the tension between a mother and a grandmother, which this arrangement can bring about often making it difficult for me to keep a balance between them in the sessions.

Of course, relationships between the women in the family can be traced in other ways too, namely through other persons who "stand behind" but who do not appear in person in the sessions. These are the men and boys: Sarah's and Chloe's dead father, who died when the girls were three and four; Peter, the little baby boy who was the first born and died very shortly before Chloe was born; Andy who was the last child to be born to Margaret and her husband before he died; and Simon, who is the youngest of Margaret's children and a son of her new relationship which has lasted many years although the couple do not live together. There are also two fathers of Olivia and Maja, who are both black men, one has been violent and abusive to Sarah and no longer has access to Olivia, the other intermittently present in Maja's life, but with an acrimonious relationship to Sarah. In the older generation the men are also described as being unhappy themselves and violent towards their wives. Margaret told me about how her mother not only had to suffer neglect when her father spent night after night in the pub, but also how he beat up his wife on several occasions. Margaret's own husband and the father to her four children (two of them dead and two alive) seriously molested her on the first night on their honeymoon and thereafter regularly. She explained that he had himself been the victim of serious physical violence from his own father and that he was mistrustful and angry. Through all of this the women, especially Margaret's mother was described as the backbone and strength for her children, and Margaret in some ways sees herself following in her footsteps holding the family together. This is a difficult task as there are other lines of rupture and conflict. Sarah has one full brother and one half-brother, but they rarely speak and when they do meet face-to-face, such as when she visits her mother and Olivia, these young men, who still live at home, leave the room and sometimes the house. At times these encounters result in verbal abuse and denigration. Margaret described that the two boys have felt that because Sarah "went off the rails", became pregnant very young and had not managed to look after Olivia on her own, and especially when she became pregnant the second time, she was taking advantage of their mother's commitment and good will. While Sarah is a sister to her two brothers, given Margaret's centrality in this relationship and the rupture between them, she is also a mother's daughter while they are mother's sons. This ambiguity Sarah shares with Olivia, because Olivia has always been difficult to parent and her grown up mother's brothers as well as Margaret's partner are described as being unsympathetic to and critical of Olivia's difficulties. Olivia is sister's daughter to her grown up uncles, but as before, considering the position of Margaret as Olivia's recognized carer, she is also a sister to them so that when there is talk of Olivia needing her own room and one of her uncles moving out of his mother's house, the difficulties and rows which this generates are similar to strong and intense sibling rivalry. In one session Margaret said that she felt that she is the only one who cares what happens to Olivia.

In the anthropological analyses which have inspired this account, for example those by Lévi-Strauss (1969), Dumont (1972) and Viveiros de Castro (2014) as well as that of Bateson in Naven,[4] men (husbands, brothers and sons) as well as women are included. Thus, in the Naven ceremony men, namely the mother's brother and the sister's son, are central actors, while women are in more shadowy positions, although mothers and sisters provide crucial channels of tension and connection between the two men. Lévi-Strauss described this as the presence of a relationship between brothers-in-law *behind* the relationship between the mother's brother and the sister's son because the mother's brother is a brother-in-law to his sister's husband (Lévi-Strauss, 1969; Viveiros de Castro, 2017) and the sister/sister-in-law is the link. In order to abandon the notion of exclusive alternatives between "sister" and "wife" as in traditional anthropological kinship theory,[5] and to convey the idea that in each relationship there is something of the other, Viveiros de Castro – quoting the analysis offered by Deleuze and Guattari – suggested that

> a given woman is in fact either my sister or my sister-in-law but "belongs precisely to both sides" [Deleuze and Guattari, 2004, p. 76] – as a sister to the side of sisters (and brothers) and as a wife on the side of wives (and husbands). Not both at once for me, but each of the two as a terminal point of the distance over which she glides... [The] one at the end of the other, like two ends of a stick in a nondecomposable space.
>
> (Viveiros de Castro, 2017, p. 132)

In other words, seen from the point of view of possibilities inherent in or emerging from the collection of relationships, which stand or exist behind any particular relationship, persons do not take up fixed positions even if they seem to do so to us. Rather they may be imbued with ambiguities of different positions as these constitute dormant or emerging possibilities. They belong to both sides in the sense that they glide over the distance between them.

Turning to the family described here in which women, rather than men, are central as is not unusual in late capitalistic single parent families, it seems to me that this describes the shifting and multiple positions which persons in the family I have described may occupy. Margaret glides over the distance between "mother" and "daughter", Sarah over "mother" and "daughter" as well as over "daughter" and "sister" and so on. Mothers, sisters and daughters and indeed anybody else in relationships have relations integral to them (Strathern, 1995, p. 165), they are reciprocally presupposed according to the conventions of the context (in any relationship there is something of the other in each), but they are also partial (each person has many such relationships) and shifting[6], and importantly they are not the same in both directions. Viveiros de Castro has explained this in the following way, providing an excellent explanation for the dynamics of schismogenesis as far as individuals are concerned:

> The crucial point here is that reciprocal presupposition determines the two poles of any duality as being equally necessary, since they are mutually conditioning, but does not thereby make them into symmetrical or equivalent poles. Inter-presupposition is an asymmetric relation: "the way is not the same in both directions".
>
> (Viveiros de Castro, 2017, p. 119)[7]

And:

> the two faces of the relational term thereby create a division internal to the terms thereby connected. Everyone becomes a double... connecter and connected are revealed to be permutable without thereby becoming redundant...
>
> (Vivieros de Castro, 2017, p. 133)

I have given a description of the family relations and kinship in this family conveying the extent of connections between persons through other persons in order to describe the multiplicity and potential openness of the possibilities these relationships offer. However, I have also described a more stubborn or repetitive theme, which I have not defined but which involves many losses and stuck entanglements. In part this was expressed in the centrality of Margaret herself, her position as a maternal figure living in late capitalism with financial and housing problems, carrying the legacy of a line of strong women with little support either from her children or from the men in her life (Edwards and Strathern, 2000). Margaret cares for everyone in her family but has herself little experience of being looked after except by her own mother. Margaret's predicament is captured well by Lambek writing about "care": "Care becomes the modality not just of kinship or memory but of engagement in the world" (Lambek, 2007, p. 238). Yet this predicament also entraps Margaret, Sarah and Olivia and also Chloe through the genealogy of their family and the lines between those who are alive, those who are dead and those who struggle all the while propped up by the conventions and constraints of social, financial and health services, housing and educational policies as well as wider kinship expectations and ideals.

Just as I began this account with a reference to schismogenesis as a way into the double-sidedness of every kinship position and the multiple possibilities of tracings of relationships this offers, I have come to think of the life, the space, the therapy room and the relationships and the processes in the family and in the work I have referred to as a "plateau", a term which Bateson used to describe as a continuing intensive stabilization rather than a climax of a schismogenic process[8] (Bateson, 1972). As has been repeated many times, Deleuze and Guattari took this term from Bateson: "We call a 'plateau' any multiplicity connected to other multiplicities by superficial underground stems in such a way as to form or extend a rhizome" (Deleuze and Guattari, 2013, p. 23). A rhizome is altogether different from a tree: "a *map and not a tracing*. Make a map not a tracing. The orchid does not reproduce the tracing of the wasp; it forms a map with the wasp, in rhizome" (Deleuze and Guattari, 2013, p. 12).

I consider that my work with families and with this family is to open up the underlying multiplicities and uncover the potentialities of the partial connections of their relationships. This is work in "the contemporary" as referred to by Rabinow and Marcus:

> if... one no longer assumes that the new is what is dominant... and that the old is somehow residual, then the question of how older and newer elements are given form and worked together, either well or poorly, becomes a significant site of inquiry. I call that site the contemporary.
>
> (Rabinow and Marcus, 2008, p. 3)

I consider the site in which therapy work described here is taking place as the "contemporary" and in it I endeavor to give meaning to the idea of what was there before, the "presentiment", and also to find that this, even though it does not yet exist, is already in action "in a different form than of its existence" (Deleuze and Guattari, 2013, p. 502). Actually here it refers to "already in action", rather than what is virtual and will come about under certain conditions (Deleuze and Guattari, 2004, p. 392). What is virtual now may thus become actual and therefore also presentiment to what becomes possible in the future. This is what I understand Deleuze to mean by the idea of immanence, "they produce while remaining in themselves" (Deleuze, quoted in May, 2005, p. 33). In the relationships between all of us in this work we could then find both stuckness as well as emerging and immanent possibilities for moving on from the stuckness.

The Ashes

A striking part of the story of this family, I think to all therapists of whatever persuasion, is the amount of death and loss (and violence) suffered by the women and especially the most central and devastating death of Chloe, symbolized by the plastic bag with her ashes in the cupboard. In Deleuzian terms I see this death as "presentiment" and already in action, and the therapy as an attempt to discover possibilities for what might emerge differently in the future, or in other words, to bring out the virtual. Chloe's death was particularly devastating because to Margaret she replaced the dead baby boy who came before her, and to Sarah, she was a close sibling and a soul mate, while at the same time the one who took her mother away from her sickbed. It is not difficult to understand why Chloe's death would be particularly difficult and painful and how her ashes have come to symbolize all losses and sufferings of the women and the family. In the UK and in Denmark we would expect a death to be mourned and, although painful, in this way to be worked through during a period of mourning, funeral and burial and regular visits to the grave thereafter. When this has not taken place and with the avoidance of speaking Chloe's name, I made the assumptions that Chloe's ashes are functioning like a fetish for this family. Generally, a fetish is known as "an object believed to procure for its owner the services of a spirit lodged within it in" (Chambers Dictionary), but for my purpose Gell (1998) offers a much more useful description of a fetish in his description of nail fetish figures from the Republic of Congo:

> An instructed person, approaching such a fetish, does not see a mere thing, a form, to which he may or may not respond aesthetically. Instead, what is seen is the visible knot, which ties together an invisible skein of relations, fanning out into social space and social time. These relations are not referred to symbolically, as if they could exist independently of their manifestation in this particular form; for these relations have produced this particular thing in its concrete factual presence; and it is because these relations exist(ed) that the fetish can exercise its judicial role.
>
> (Gell, 1998, p. 62)

I would substitute "judicial" for "emotional" without in any way diminishing the social function of Chloe's ashes for this family. I also follow Latour's account in making no particular sharp distinction between "facts" which are thought to be real and "fetishes" which are thought to be imaginary (Latour, 2010).[9] In this way Gell's idea of the fetish beautifully picks up Deleuze's and Guattari's point that "Symbols and fetishes are manifestations of desiring machines" (Deleuze and Guattari, 2004, p. 200). They further write:

> A machine works according to the previous intercommunications of its structure and positioning of its parts, but does not set itself into place any more than it forms or reproduces itself... in one way or another the machine and desire thus remain in an extrinsic relationship, either because desire appears as an effect determined by a system of mechanical causes, or because the machine is itself a system of means in terms of the aims of desire.
>
> (Deleuze and Guattari, 2004, p. 312)[10]

I venture to argue that the centrality of women and care in the family and the way, as I have shown, this is inherent in the relationships between them invests and is invested in by the desire in this family to have no more losses, to have no more conflicts and "to be an ordinary family", as often expressed by Sarah in our therapy sessions. This has psychological and emotional effects, which in turn function as an investment in social and political expectations about the role of women in contemporary UK white English/Irish working class society. Therefore, in the ongoing therapy it is, and will be, difficult to move on or to find vitality without thinking about this machine manifested in Chloe's ashes. I have already explained that I had the idea that somehow Chloe's ashes in the cupboard prevented the family relations and the communication becoming unstuck and that Margaret did not agree. However, perhaps Sarah, by not wanting to talk about Chloe, showed me that the ashes did have something of a taboo about them and that therefore there was a feeling of ambivalence about whether or not Chloe's ashes protected or hindered the ongoing relationships in the family.

Understanding

To return to the opening statements of this chapter I can now ask: How do I understand the continuing presence of the ashes in the cupboard and how might I proceed or indeed live in the therapy work with this family? Do I consider the ashes in the cupboard a manifestation of pathology and in this way follow a long tradition of psychoanalytically influenced thinking about unresolved loss and mourning in Western psychology? Margaret rejected this when she told me that other mothers too keep their dead children's ashes indicating, I thought, that my point of view is that of someone who has not experienced the loss of a child myself and therefore I cannot know or make a judgment about it. She is of course correct, I am different from her, from a different class, from a different country and culture, with different experiences of work, and I have not lost a child. Do I then consider that the ashes as a manifestation of a desiring machine are locking the family into particular socially determined (and emotional) types of familial relationships, which cannot be changed without challenging their very rationale of existence? Do I consider that the existence of the ashes in the airing cupboard is inevitable, perhaps like a fetish even protective, and that this is how this family must live? And under what circumstances would this give rise to something new, what Deleuze and Guattari refer to as a line of flight (Guattari, 2016)? And what part could I play? Would I be able to approach the ashes and the relationships manifested in them from a position of "reality in parenthesis", in which,

> following this explanatory path, the observer becomes aware that each domain of reality is a domain of entities constituted in the explanation of

his or her praxis of living with the operational coherences of his or her
praxis of living.

(Maturana, 1988, p. 39)

This point has often been debated in social anthropology and especially in
relation to the Oedipus complex (Malinowski, 1929; Obeyesekere, 1990;
Spiro, 1987), but also recently with respect to how to understand a fetish. The
debate has centered around what has come to be referred to as "the Ontological Turn" in social anthropology (Holbraad and Pedersen, 2017; Viveiros de
Castro, 2014) and the debate has something to say, as does so much of
anthropology, about how systemic psychotherapists may approach their clients, their own work and their own lives. I shall focus on the interchange
between Eduardo Viveiros de Castro and David Graeber, another well-known
anthropologist, activist and critic of capitalism (Graeber, 2015; Viveiros de
Castro, 2014).

In Graeber's ethnographic work with the Merina (Graeber, 1996), a hail
charm, referred to as Ravololona, was considered to have the power to
stop the hail, which often ruined Malagasy crops. Viveiros accuses Graeber of denying the legitimacy of this Merina view, when he says that he,
Graeber, does not believe that the Ravololona can really stop the hail and
that the explanation for the Ravololona is that the fetish is a projection of
social relations of some sort, in the same way as I quoted Gell to argue
above and in which I might consider Chloe's ashes to be a manifestation
of relations in the family described here. Graeber's analysis is more complex and radical and I have a good deal of respect for his idea that fetishes
invite a disjunction between what people say they believe and how they
act,[11] just as Margaret rejected the stuckness in the family having anything
to do with the ashes, but still acted as if it was of utmost importance that
they stay in the cupboard. Graeber argues that this paradox between belief
and action is typical of moments of social creativity and of politics.
Viveiros de Castro claims that thinking about the Ravololona in this way
amounts to Graeber trying to make his arguments "behind the natives
back" because the Merina would not agree with his analysis. I shall not
pursue the arguments of the debate here as these are both extensive and
technical; suffice to say that the "Ontological Turn"[12] refers to the position
of Viveiros and others, that

ontological questions are political questions insofar as they come into
existence only in the context of friction and divergence between concepts,
given, I stress the polysemic value of this word, given the absolute absence
of any exterior or superior arbiter. Ontological differences, to get the
point are political because they imply a situation of war- not a war of
words, as per linguistic turn, but an ongoing war of *worlds*.

(Viveiros de Castro, 2014, p. 11; emphasis in original)[13]

The Ontological Turn is "the turn of the native, the act of making room for the other... the obligation of letting the natives whoever they are, have it ontologically speaking their own way" (Viveiros de Castro, 2014, p. 10).

Correspondence

Graeber questioned Viveiros de Castro's idea of "ontology" as "way of being" or simply "being", arguing that the more standard definition of the term "ontology" is "*talk* about being or life" (Graeber, 2015, p. 15). This difference maps onto the difference between "parenthesis" or "without parenthesis" (Maturana, 1988) and speaks directly to how systemic psychotherapists conduct therapy through "being" as well as through "talking about being". Nevertheless, to be honest, these two positions leave a gap for me too between what I might say I want to do and what I might do. How do I escape my own ontology, whether this is my life or my talk about my life? I know that I may have trouble distinguishing my "talk about my life" from "my life" as I already demonstrated in my leap to assuming that the ashes in the cupboard keep the family stuck and that Chloe cannot come to life again without these being taken care of in the – for me and in my experience – expected way.

Could I think about this differently? The Mothers of the Plaza de Mayo movement from Argentina and their struggle in encountering loss may help me (Robben, 2000).[14] This movement arose after the events during the Argentine dirty war from 1976 to 1983 in which thousands of people, many of them young, were disappeared by the military regime, and the reactions of the mothers of disappeared children. Most disappeared were killed within a few days or weeks after their capture, but parents were deliberately left in the dark, not knowing whether their children were alive or dead. Most were taken from their homes at night while families were sleeping and for the parents this questioned their ability to protect their children and children's trust in their parents. The continuing lack of knowledge about whether the children were dead or alive made funerals and ordinary processes of mourning and grief impossible. This led to a now famous demonstration by the mothers of the disappeared against the disappearances of their sons and daughters. The mothers demonstrated every week wearing nappies as headscarves and became known as the Mothers of the Plaza de Mayo across the world. The disappearances are shameful events with unimaginable suffering which continued over many years, and the action of the Mothers was a powerful demonstration of the intersection of the Mothers' political actions with their grief and anguish. I am interested in the events after the military junta fell in 1983 and when mass graves of the victims were identified and reopened. According to Robben the majority of the Mothers condemned the exhumations of the graves on the grounds that these were part of a government scheme to have the Mothers accept (and therefore participate in) the death of the disappeared. The Mothers demanded that those responsible should be brought to trial first. The Mothers expressed it in these terms:

> In many respects it was like this: my children had given birth to me... If they are not here, then I have to be them, shout for them, vindicate them with honesty and return if even a small piece of life to them. They are my rallying cries, in this fatigue that maybe nobody can understand but which always recuperates itself, they are in my head and in my body, in everything I do. I believe that their absence has left me forever pregnant.
> (Sanchez, 1985, pp. 74–75, quoted in Robben, 2000, p. 93)

The Mothers had no ashes, while Margaret has the bag of Chloe's ashes in the cupboard. However, might Margaret, the ashes machine and the over-deter-mination of women's care in the family I have described here share this outlook with the Mothers? That is to say, is Margaret an embodiment of Chloe (and her other children) in such a way that the exhausting theme of devoted care continually "recuperates" itself and by its very process reproduces the situation giving space for life? A funeral for Chloe would mean that Chloe would need no more care, or not as much care, and perhaps bury Margaret's pain of loss and separation, instead of, as I had so clumsily put it, bringing her "to life again". It is interesting to note that eventually exhumations and reburial did take place in Argentina on a wide scale with both political and psychological significance and the Mothers transferred the suffering of their children to the suffering of all victims and to radical political ideas.

How then may I position myself in my future work with this family? I have tried to show that by jumping to the conclusion that Chloe's ashes need a burial I am traversing too much territory in one go, because this direct con-nection in some way colonizes by pointing only in one direction. A funeral and a mourning period may still be needed but as with the Mothers there will be some steps before that. I am sure that another quality is needed and again Deleuze and Guattari are helpful, if not in giving direction, in providing inspiration. I am thinking here of their thoughts on the "smooth" and the "striated" (Deleuze and Guattari, 2013, pp. 551–582).

> Smooth space is filled by events or haecceities, far more than by formed and perceived things. It is a space of affects, more than one of properties. It is *haptic* rather than optical perception. Whereas the striated forms organise matter, in the smooth materials signal forces and serve as symptoms for them. It is an intensive rather than an extensive, space, one of distances, not of measures and properties.
> (Deleuze and Guattari, 2013, p. 557, emphasis in the original)

Striated space can be exemplified by regular, rectilinear intersections as in woven fabric, whereas smooth space can be exemplified by felt, since felt is a mixture of entangled fibers made of wool and can be stretched and formed in all directions, as in those little felt figures children play with. Any analysis or process necessarily passes between smooth and striated spaces giving way to each other. It seems to me that therapy can also be characterized as smooth and striated and that the most difficult bit for the therapist is to notice, or to be in the smooth space. In the events I have described here I did not always manage, but I did develop a realization of what I needed in order to be in a smooth space. I needed to get close enough to be in touch with the partial, multiple and double quality of all kinship and relations in which "it is not the same in both directions" in order to realize the potential of new possibilities for the life of this family. "Getting close to" in this sense resonates with what Ingold has referred to as a "discipline of correspondence" (Ingold, 2017, p. 24) which he defines as "co-operating with one's work" (Ingold, 2013, p. 128) or the "attentional movement in which the movement resonates with the things to which it attends" (p. 18). Ingold offers the image of "taking another by the hand", and Dewey's notion of "having things in common being not a prerequisite but an outcome of communication" (Dewey, 1966, p. 4, quoted in Ingold, 2017, p. 14). Ingold explains:

> To have in common is not to look inside ourselves, to regress to a set of baseline attributes with which we are similarly endowed from the start, but to reach out to others who are – at least initially – different from us.
>
> (Ingold, 2017, pp. 14–15)

Perhaps my own experiences of being cared for by a grandmother and of the conflict between my mother and grandmother predisposed me to understand the events in this family, or perhaps these experiences stood in the way. Either way these are experiences to which I could get near. I agree with both Graeber and Viveiros de Castro, whose points of view do not seem to me to be contradictory. The ashes are a manifestation of a paradox, namely that through them the kinship relations in this family are held together while at the same time straining towards another reality, that persons stand in multiple positions as well as partial connections in relation to each other, and that these connections are not the same in both directions. I imagine that Bateson would have agreed with both Graeber and Viveiros de Castro that such a paradox is a precondition for creativity, a creativity of the contemporary to which the therapist may contribute if she is able to "co-operate with her work". I believe that my mistake became the beginning of a process through which my understanding changed from considering the ashes as a sign of stuckness and something inhibiting, to seeing them as a sign of the continuous and unfolding care, which the women in this family engage in despite the adversity in their past, current and perhaps future lives. I came to appreciate and respect the vitality of the ashes as their presence offered the possibility of going in both directions and in this I was helped by the Mothers of the Plaza de Mayo.

Concluding Remarks

I began this chapter by pointing out that Gilles Deleuze and his colleague Felix Guattari rarely speak of "culture", but that this does not mean that they do not address this aspect of social contexts. On the contrary, it sometimes appears that they are inspired by the way things and relationships emerge in social contexts, which cannot be described as capitalist. We may say the same about Bateson, even though his collaboration with psychiatric colleagues in some way may have forced him to be blunt, he never wrote of "culture" as something essentialized, which stands apart from any interaction, communication, dialogue or apprehension. "Culture" is never outside. What is outside is "another" situated in all his or her relationships and social, political and economic contexts, ways of doing and understanding the world, and the extent of this "outsidedness" is a matter of scale. The issue is, though, always there. As Foucault observed it has been increasingly located in the "language from which the subject is excluded" (Foucault, 1987, p. 15) as in "thoughts from the outside". This is why I began this chapter with the question: How do I understand someone else? Perhaps a silly question as this is the bread and butter of psychotherapy. Nevertheless, perhaps we have neglected to make a thorough re-assessment of this task, particularly as social processes and the involvement of the State in our mental health service structures, certainly in the UK, increasingly dictate the limits, forms and structures of our encounters with those who ask us for help.

I have attempted to address two issues in this chapter. First, I have indicated that in order to take "difference" seriously I suggest that we look inside the concept of "relationship" and this takes us to an appreciation of the implications of beginning not just with an assumption of a type of "unified personhood" but to a concept of a person derived from other prior and contemporary relationships, someone who therefore already is a multiplicity. In this way a person occupies multiple positions, "gliding" over these according to context, the relationship in question and to what is available. What is available is always also a multiplicity. Perhaps there is a tendency to forget this when we systemic psychotherapists work with genograms rather than kinship. Second, I have tried to show how this view opens up more space and more hopefulness about how I, the therapist, may find ways of understanding the predicament of a family through the concepts and thought which they themselves put into practice. This last point is in part a result of taking seriously that my relationship with those who come to see me is equally partial and not the same in both directions. Yet, in any encounter, in any relationship, there is an exchange in which there is something, words, things, feelings, glances and gestures, passed to me from the other and the other way around. Systemic psychotherapists have of course always known that, but I think we have often been seduced by what *we identify* as the appearance of a connection or a difference.

The Ontolgial Turn suggests that what differs is not just epistemologies, i.e. how we access and understand what there is, but also that "reality" itself can be different to different people and in different situations. In this way there is not just one, colonial, objective ontology, but many ontologies. I have tried to show how seriously "difference" is taken in this approach, and for this reason alone I think this approach merits the attention of systemic psychotherapists. In my work with the family described here, taking difference seriously meant that I could not assume that each of the six women in the encounter, including myself, occupied only one position at any one time. Rather, we all took up different relational aspects of ourselves on the one hand echoing social, political, linguistic and kinship relationships, what Deleuze calls "extensive", of real contemporary contexts. On the other hand, these relational aspects contained within them some possibilities for going forward, the virtual or what Deleuze refers to as the "intensive". The virtual is therefore greater than the real, and actualizing the virtual involves selecting from the real as well as limiting it. The tension between these two processes, I think, was played out for me in the thinking about "the ashes". My way of understanding "the ashes" left in the cupboard for so many years as a stuckness missed the point of what they were for the women in this family. I was helped by the example of the Mothers of the Plaza de Mayo to understand other possibilities. I did not bring up the Mothers of the Plaza de Mayo with this family, nor did we talk very much more about the ashes again. Perhaps the change happened in me in-between the two sessions, which I have described earlier in this chapter, and it has taken some time for me to process this. I have not come to accept Margaret's view about the ashes as a kind of indigenous understanding far removed from my own. Rather I have come to understand the vitality of these ashes and the possibilities they open up. One of these was "continuous care", and this concept allowed for a correspondence to emerge between my understanding and theirs. This correspondence was not a matter of me holding my concept of "mourning" nor their concept of "care" tight, but a matter of me accepting that for this family at this moment "care" was a perspective, or, paraphrasing Viveiros de Castro, "care" in this family was itself an "implication of the very concept of perspective" (Viveiros de Castro, 2013, p. 499). To search for the perspectives of those with whom I work is perhaps as much as any systemic psychotherapist can hope for.

Notes

1 This turn of phrase derives from Foucault's discussion of Maurice Blanchot's writing on the topic of literature. Foucault contrasts the interiority of saying "I speak" with the exteriority of literature in which "the subject that speaks is less the responsible agent of a discourse… than a non-existence in whose emptiness the unending outpouring of language uninterruptedly continues" (Foucault, 1987, p. 11). This is a thought which stands outside subjectivity "setting its limits as though from without" (Foucault, 1987, p. 15). These ideas are well known from Foucauldian discourse analysis.

2

> For Oedipus to be occupied, it is not enough that it be a limit or a displaced represented in the system of representation; it must *migrate* to the heart of this system and itself come to occupy the position of the representative of desire These conditions, inseperable from the paralogisms of the unconscious, are realized in the capitalist formation; furthermore they imply certain archaisms from the imperial barbarian formations- in particular, the position of the transcendent object.
>
> (Deleuze and Guattari, 2004, p.194, italics in original)

3 Filiation refers to being a child of a specific parent. It implies "the recognition of four sets of relationships: those between the woman and man who engendered the child, between the child and its mother, the child and its father, and between siblings, that is children of the same parents" (Holy, 1996).

Traditionally anthropologists contrast this with "alliance" which refers to an exchange of partners between exclusive groups. Alliance theory is associated with Lévi-Strauss's groundbreaking structuralist work on marriage systems (Lévi-Strauss, 1969). These definitions are somewhat strained in the context of contemporary kinship (same-sex marriage, IVF etc.). However, the main point in traditional kinship studies was to flag up the distinction between the biosocial and emotional life of "the family" and its legal, economic and political dimensions. Along with other later anthropologists Deleuze and Guattari offer a critique of this distinction when they suggest that "A kinship system only appears closed to the extent that it is severed from the political and economic references that keep it open, and that make alliance something other than an arrangement of matrimonial classes and filiative lineages" (Deleuze and Guattari, 2004, p. 162).

4 The central relationship around which the Naven ceremony revolves beautifully illustrates the point made by Deleuze and Guattari because this is both filiation and alliance: filiation because a sister's son traces his relationship to his mother's brother through his mother and alliance because this is expressed in the relationship between a man and his sister's husband.

5 In Lévi-Straussian structuralism this is referred to as "the atom of kinship", in this way recognizing the biosocial in any familial relationship.

6 Deleuze refers to "presupposition" as a return to "a world in which all previous identities have been abolished and dissolved" (Deleuze, 1994, p. 52). Relations are therefore not reciprocal by way of imitation or analogy. They are generative of a new way of being that is a function of influences rather than resemblances.

7 See also the opening of Ingold's 2017 paper, which starts with the words "Let me take you by the hand" (Ingold, 2017, p. 9).

8 This refers to the chapter "Bali: The value system of a steady state" in *Steps to An Ecology of Mind* (Bateson, 1972).

9 The term is often thought of as derogatory.

10 There is no space here to elaborate on Deleuze's and Guattari's use of the terms "mechanical" or "machine". For further reading see May (2005) and Nichterlein and Morss (2017).

11 Graeber includes commodity fetishism in his critique.

12 Graeber claims that "ontology" refers to a discourse about "being" or "mode of existence" whereas Viveiros and colleagues of the same persuasion use the term to refer to "a way of being itself" (Graeber, 2015, p. 15).

13 This is a reference to the earlier so-called "linguistic turn" in the social sciences, in which researchers assumed the primacy of language and acknowledged that their descriptions and data reflected the researcher's own established use of language.

14 I am grateful to Felicity Tyson for bringing this paper to my attention.

References

Bateson, G. (1958). *Naven: The Culture of the Iatmul People of New Guinea as Revealed through a Study of the "Naven" Ceremonial*. London: Wildwood House.

Bateson, G. (1972). *Steps to An Ecology of Mind: Collected Essays in Anthropology, Psychiatry, Evolution and Epistemology*. London: Jason Aronson.

Bialecki, J. (2018). Deleuze. In F. Stein, S. Lazar, M. Candea, H. Diemberger, J. Robbins, A. Sanchez and R. Stasch (eds), *The Cambridge Encyclopedia of Anthropology*. Cambridge: Cambridge University Press. http://doi.org/10.29164/18deleuze

Bohannan, L. and Bohannan, P. (1953). *The Tiv of Central Nigeria*. London: International African Institute.

Bourdieu, P. (1998). *Practical Reason*. Cambridge: Polity Press.

Deleuze, G. (1994). *Difference and Repetition*. London: Bloomsbury.

Deleuze, G. and Guattari, F. (2004). *Anti-Oedipus: Capitalism and Schizophrenia*. London: Continuing International Publishing Group (First published 1972).

Deleuze, G. and Guattari, F. (1991). *What is Philosophy?* New York: Columbia University Press.

Deleuze, G. and Guattari, F. (2013). *A Thousand Plateaus*. London: Bloomsbury Academic (First published 1987).

Dewey, J. (1966). *Democracy and Education: An Introduction to the Philosophy of Education*. New York: The Free Press.

Dumont, L. (1972). *Homo Hierarchicus: The Caste System and Its Implications*. London: Paladin.

Edwards, J. and Strathern, M. (2000). Including our own. In J. Carsten (ed.), *Cultures of Relatedness: New Approaches in the Study of Kinship*. Cambridge: Cambridge University Press.

Foucault, M. (1987). Maurice Blanchot: The thought from outside. In *Foucault/Blanchot*. New York. Zone Books.

Gell, A. (1998). *Art and Agency: An Anthropological Theory*. Oxford: The Clarendon Press.

Graeber, D. (1996). Love magic and political morality in Central Madagascar, 1875–1990. *Gender and History*, 8 (3), 416–439.

Graeber, D. (2015). Radical alterity is just another way of saying "reality": A reply to Eduardo Viveiros de Castro. *HAU: Journal of Ethnographic Theory*, 5(2), 1–41.

Griaule, M. (1965). *Conversations with Ogotemmeli: An Introduction to Dogon Religious Ideas*. Oxford: Oxford University Press (First published 1948).

Guattari, F. (2016). *Lines of Flight: For Another World of Possibilities*. London: Bloomsbury Academic.

Harries-Jones, P. (1995). *A Recursive Vision: Ecological Understanding and Gregory Bateson*. Toronto: Toronto University Press.

Holbraad, M. and Pedersen, M.A. (2017). *The Ontological Turn: An Anthropological Exposition*. Cambridge: Cambridge University Press.

Holy, L. (1996). *Anthropological Perspectives on Kinship*. London: Pluto Press.

Ingold, T. (2013). *Making: Anthropology, Archaeology, Art and Architecture*. Abingdon: Routledge.

Ingold, T. (2017). On human correspondence. *Journal of the Royal Anthropological Institute*, 23(1), 9–27.

Krause, I.-B. (2007). Reading Naven: Towards the integration of culture in systemic psychotherapy. *Human Systems*, 18, 112–125.

Krause, I.-B. (2012). Culture and the reflexive subject in systemic psychotherapy. In I.-B. Krause (ed.), *Mutual Perspective: Culture and Reflexivity in Systemic Psychotherapy*. London: Karnac Books.

Lambek, M. (2007). The cares of Alice Alder: Recuperating kinship and history in Switzerland. In J. Carsten (ed.), *Ghosts of Memory: Essays on Remembrance and Relatedness*. Oxford: Blackwell Publishing.

Latour, B. (2010). *On the Modern Cult of the Factish Gods*. Durham, NC: Duke University Press.

Lévi-Strauss, C. (1969). *The Elementary Structures of Kinship*. Boston, MA: Beacon Press.

Malinowski, B. (1929). *The Sexual Life of Savages in North-Western Melanesia*. London: Routledge & Kegan Paul.

Maturana H. (1988). Reality: The search for objectivity or the quest for a compelling argument. *Irish Journal of Psychology*, 9(1), 25–82.

May, T. (2005). *Gilles Deleuze: An Introduction*. Cambridge: Cambridge University Press.

Nichterlein, M. and Morss, J.R. (2017). *Deleuze and Psychology: Philosophical Provocations and Psychological Practices*. Abingdon: Routledge.

Obeyesekere, G. (1990). *The Work of Culture: Symbolic Transformation in Psychoanalysis and Anthropology*. Chicago, IL: The The University of Chicago Press.

Rabinow, P. and Marcus, G.E. (2008). *Designs for an Anthropology of the Contemporary*. Durham, NC: Duke University Press.

Robben, A.C.G.M. (2000). The assault on basic trust: Disappearance, protest, and reburial in Argentina. In A.C.G.M. Robben and M.M. Suarez-Orozco (eds), *Cultures under Siege: Collective Violence and Trauma*. Cambridge: Cambridge University Press.

Spiro, M. (1987). *Culture and Human Nature: Theoretical Papers of Melford E. Spiro*. Chicago, IL: The University of Chicago Press.

Strathern, M. (1995). The nice thing about culture is that everybody has it. In M. Strathern (ed.), *Shifting Contexts. Transformations in Anthropological Knowledge*, pp. 153–176. London: Routledge.

Strathern, M. (2004). *Partial Connections*, updated edn. Oxford: Altamira Press.

Turner, V. (2000). An Ndembu doctor in practice. In R. Littlewood and S. Dein (eds), *Cultural Psychiatry and Medical Anthropology*. London: The Athlone Press (First published 1964).

Viveiros de Castro, E. (2013). The relative native. *HAU: Journal of Ethnographic Theory*, 3(3), 473–502.

Viveiros de Castro, E. (2014). Who is afraid of the ontological wolf? Some comments on an ongoing anthropological debate. CUSAS Annual Marilyn Strathern Lecture. Cambridge, 30 May.

Viveiros de Castro, E. (2017). *Cannibal Metaphysics*. London: University of Minnesota Press.

Watzlawick, P., Bavelas, J.B. and Jackson, D.J. (1967). *Pragmatics of Human Communication: A Study of Interactional Patterns, Pathologies and Paradoxes*. New York: W.W. Norton & Company.

Chapter 5

Getting Sick from Psychotherapy

Our Co-Responsibility in Unintended and Undesired Outcomes

Umberta Telfener

Introduction

When I agreed to contribute to this book, I was very curious about my co-authors' interest in Deleuze, for our shared positioning against the linguistic turn and for the similarities that I felt were present between us. We share some of the views proposed in these chapters: symptoms as indicators; interpretation as a risky attitude that freezes the process and assumes the hegemony of a central signifier; the need to create new relationships and territories in order to bring out the virtual; considering "becoming" as the process on which to concentrate. We share the idea that things are rhizomatically interconnected. We are interested in how experience can be transformed, in how events are unique, in how difference makes the ordinary possible. We all recognize the importance of generating singular encounters in a process of small gestures. We reject neutrality, objectivity and Truth with a capital T.

Heinz von Foerster has been my mentor, the most beloved and significant teacher in my professional development. He taught me wonder; he insisted that understanding is an environment one enters, a process in which we participate as part of life, an emotion in reality. He insisted on singularities and novelties, on the new as a doubt that breaks the status quo and destabilizes the self, on ruptures that propose lines of flight. He described possibilities as multiplicities of differential relationships, always engaged in the context. He ascribed importance to unpredictability and to the effort to promote windows of opportunity through attention to movement and connections.

Deleuze, von Foerster and Bateson, as well as Maturana and Varela, are all philosophers of difference and possibility, thought creators, divergent thinkers interested in investigating worlds of shifting ecologies, fascinated by inclusion, instability, and what is in movement. They are generative thinkers interested in newness and evolution. They all state that unnoticed differences and relationships among things and ideas determine new lines of flight: they believe there are many potentialities in every moment, many possible configurations. They are irreverent masters of freedom, and all of them have made room for the creation of new possible worlds.

DOI: 10.4324/9780429437410-5

Within our systemic epistemology, the therapist does not know any better or any more than the client. Her[1] theories, her hypotheses, her comments are neither true nor false; they are plausible exactly as those of the client. What differentiates the two positions is that the professional's hypotheses belong to a different order, not at the content level of what one thinks, or at the first-order level of "understanding", but rather at the second-order level of "understanding our understanding" and "knowing about knowing". I am proposing a multiple positioning, not so much of different kinds of *capta* (Laing, 1961, proposed calling data "*capta*" since they are not given once and for all, but are chosen by the subject), but rather a manifold point of view which combines: 1) the consideration of the context in which we are acting; 2) a study of the newly emerged therapeutic system that includes the professional, the client, and all the significant relationships that embrace them; 3) the observation of the asymmetrical but equal relationship established within the becoming ecology; 4) a reflection on the generativity of the process, on the poetics that emerges from what can be proposed, said, and done in the therapy room.

The professional needs a broader awareness, not about herself but about the relational aspects that connect everyone and the dance[2] she is performing with the other(s). Becoming is a change in the way of relating to the habitual elements of our existence. Clients bring us an explicit, organized and repetitive narrative that is making them suffer, and we propose redefinitions and actions, through a self-organizing process, recursive, that includes all the participants interacting, including other professionals who deal with the same system. The clinical work has to do with finding our way in this multitude of definitions and relationships, reflecting on each one's participation as a way to make new connections appear. We ask ourselves: What lines of flight will emerge? How can we perturb the system that is already in constant evolution, through our listening, speaking, acting, laughing, sharing together?

It is from this co-creative process that an evolutive process emerges – involving *all* the people and agencies who rotate around a life script (the problem-determined system), consciously aware of their common dance or just attentive to the others, with the hope more than the need of collaborating. The constructivist professional cannot avoid values. She needs to take a political[3] position (Pakman, 2018) and assume responsibility for connecting with others through actions, working with the other's subjectivity and with her own, with the ideas and relationships personified in the dance, which is an active action. The therapeutic job is no longer a technical one. Therapy always implies an ethical, an aesthetic, as well as a political, stance.

The Aim of This Chapter

Within a systemic, circular, participatory epistemology, nothing is good or harmful in itself. It can be defined either one way or the other only within a relationship and a context. Successes or failures do not depend unilaterally on the clinician or on the client. They are generated within the story of their connection and of their reciprocal encounter. Good results in practice are not guaranteed by theories or techniques or by their correct application; nor does a correct use of epistemological presuppositions and clinical operations guarantee satisfying results. Clinical interventions emerge from participating in a shared reality within a collaborative, co-responsible and dialogical context. Successes and failures in psychotherapy and communal interventions emerge from the coordination of coordination of actions and meanings. It therefore becomes necessary for the professional to join the dance as an active participant and operate from a stance in which she recognizes a multiple positioning towards knowledge, always honoring complexity.

Why did I choose this subject for my contribution to this book? Why did I choose to write about the risks inherent our work? Because I think this subject is consistent with and complementary to the themes addressed by my co-authors. Because therapy is too often taken for granted and thought of as a linear determined process within a "cult of the therapeutic" (Kinman, 2017): in this case each therapy shows results; there are no differences between models and the people who perform them and therapy becomes a much-valued process, reified, with a priori rules and trivial relationships. Because Western professionals tend to verify the process of psychotherapy instead of falsifying it: they prefer to consider everything they do useful and correct until proven otherwise. Because, if therapy is a second-order operation – as I state as a premise – we need to reflect on the observing system (von Foerster, 1984) and on the process we facilitate, rather than on the observed system alone, the system which asked for help. Because we face unpredictable problems and undeterminable situations and we can find ourselves stuck in blueprints that perpetrate chronicity and are not generative and we therefore need to reflect on such occurrences without fear. Therapy can produce a change of regimes, can free life from its stagnation. We need to pay attention to small gestures and identify new components through the creation of new relationships and territories.

I will speak about the possibility that the process we create leads to chronicity and collusion, to a stuck script that does not open up new possibilities. I will address the risk of iatrogenic risk as the possibility that an intervention ends in an aggravation and that we become Doctor Homeostat (Hoffman, 2012), that the process results in a deterioration of emotions, relationships and quality of life. Therapy needs instead to continue to be a generative space, in which new information emerges into places it did not inhabit before, where we connect with something different from ourselves, entering into proximity zones with the other(s). A generative space where we need to invent and discover assemblages of relations, cooperating with our own work.

The practice I will describe involves designing unstable maps, mapping processes and relations, playing, the capacity to get involved, to risk and improvise. It implicates a becoming, co-creating, a setting in which each participant has the possibility of self-transformation, of passing from one state to another. As Deleuze proposes, analyzing *Moby-Dick*, "becoming in a middle zone", the possibility, through the encounter/confrontation/clash between subjectivities, of feeling and getting emotional in relation to the other, having abandoned one's own unique identity, finding oneself in a dimension that is different from the one each had started from; being chained together in a relationship that transformed each one, after the encounter. Becoming means being overwhelmed by the vortex of a transformation. What Deleuze calls *deterritorialize* (out-land), an experiential process, a "mapping that is always detachable, connectable, reversible, modifiable, and has multiple entrance ways and it exists and has its own lines of flight"[4] (Deleuze and Guattari, 1987, p. 72), a plane of immanence to extend the territory one is in by perceiving areas of intensity, by giving up some of one's boundaries.

The lack of recognition of these difficulties on the part of the professional, the acceptance of everything that emerges in the dance between the clinician and the client, can lead to the *unintended outcomes* I wish to speak about. Luckily, we also participate together in the wisdom of life and utilize our creative generative power to contribute to the process; we participate in what is happening and open up "the underlying multiplicities".

How much time must pass before we consider a situation worsened? According to clinical research, professionals with a psychodynamic orientation need around 14 months, since their paradigm states the possibility of the client's getting worse in order to get better; cognitive therapists wait six to eight months before acknowledging impasse. Systemic professionals tend to intervene after a very short time, since we do not theorize hurt as embedded in the therapeutic process, and we are usually imprinted to a brief processual kind of work (Bianciardi and Telfener, 2014). The usual reasons cited to explain any block in the therapeutic process are mainly attributed to the severity of the clients' personality or his/her problems, rarely to the therapeutic relationship, and almost never to the clinician's actions. For us systems evolve naturally. Intervening can thus slow down or even block this evolutive process. In these cases, the professional – monitoring the evolution of a co-evolution in the co-defined process – senses, through her feelings and reflections, that there is no progress, or that the process has become harmful, since interactions and emotions can hurt.

Humans as Unpredictable, Context as Undeterminable

It is Heinz von Foerster, among others, who invites us to a continuous imperfection and incompleteness, to a constant temporariness, to the awareness of not being final. Believing that sensory experience and action were central to living, von Foerster stated that learning to live and psychotherapy are two processes that could proceed in parallel, since they both require similar operations and isomorphic processes. Psychotherapy is a territory in which stories told are not connected to truth but to a process of coherence and adaptation. The Anthropos is immersed in a constant process of becoming.

Gödel's Incompleteness Theorem, Heisenberg's Uncertainty Principle, and Gill's Undeterminable Principle have opened up to an "epistemology of ignorance" proposed by my mentor: "Moreover, it is a contradiction because epistemology means 'theory of knowledge' and how could you have a 'theory of knowledge of ignorance'?" von Foerster asks.

> Indeed, it is precisely this sort of paradoxical situation of an epistemology and, on the other hand, of ignorance that moved me to address this very problem. It has appeared to me lately that we do not grasp the tremendous amount of ignorance on which our knowledge sits, like a small speck on the top of a gigantic iceberg.
>
> (von Foerster, 1992, p. 61)

It is difficult to adapt to one's ignorance. It is not purely by chance that our culture gives as synonyms for this stance "illiteracy", "incompetence", "incapability", "inexperience". The two forms of ignorance about which von Foerster speaks are not negatively declined and are caused by *undeterminables*, which occur when one cannot determine the properties of a system, and *undecidables*, which occur when one cannot decide whether a proposition is true or false and we cannot know the answer to a question. He proposed *lethology* [5] as the calculus of unknowable: how to deal with humans that are in principle undeterminable and how to answer questions that are in principle undecidable.

According to von Foerster, the world is organized by *trivial* and *non-trivial* machines. The first ones fit exactly to the notion we have of a machine. They do the thing they are supposed to do. The result is always the same (cars, toasters and computers would be trivial machines). Then there are non-trivial machines: when they have completed a particular procedure, they change their internal operation system into another one. If one proposes the same problem again, the non-trivial machine does not come up with the same answer. It gives a different answer, according to the different internal rules which have inevitably changed. The latter are desiring devices, history dependent, unpredictable and analytically undeterminable[6] (human beings, the immune system, the universe).

Operating at the level of knowing/not knowing is very different from operating at a second-order level (knowing that one knows, knowing that one does not know); in the second case, the relationship with knowledge is influenced by our beliefs about knowledge itself, and we are pressed to analyze the categories adopted, the metaphors chosen, the process which has emerged. We get away from the content and reflect on the process. Making a diagnosis, for example, implies making an a priori categorization, using knowledge as the main construct in a first-order manner. The risk is that of acting as if concepts were set in stone, of taking the categories for granted instead of questioning each concept.

Similarly, the medical model defines the sick person as "ignorant about health and illness" and needs him/her to be compliant with the directives of doctors, "the experts", those who have often first-order solutions, applying standard procedures. The systemic model, on the other hand, implies that the clients are experts in their own lives, while the professionals are experts in change processes: they can hypothesize that the presenting problem will evolve but are ignorant of the solutions the system will choose. The medical model operates at a first-order mode and follows generalized procedures always the same while us systemic psychotherapists are organized by singularities and operations over operations, constant reflections on the operations we propose.

Professionals need to think about the categories they have utilized, to project themselves into a possible generative future, to have plans and desires, to imagine that systems inevitably evolve. We participate in a multitude of *self-organizing systems* able to modify themselves in a non-deterministic and unpredictable mode. Therapy becomes a self-organizing system able to give shape to the interactive reality, in order to guarantee the maintenance of its organization, to guarantee the client as a client and the clinician as a clinician.

If we forget that humans are unpredictable and context undeterminable – a prejudiced statement itself – we risk falling into the field we create with our clients and become static: we buy their premises, fall into their usual relational processes and adapt to the behaviors that organize their lives. We also collapse into our own patterns and prejudices. If we do not organize a second-order process that involves us and allows us to reflect on our reflections, we risk reifying homeostatic patterns even if we conduct therapy in a formally "perfect" manner. We need to reflect on the patterns in which we participate and the ideas and emotions that we share.

I will describe some unintended outcomes through some different cases in which therapeutic blocks occurred.

Biagio and Anna come for couples therapy with me. He has a degree in history and works as a blacksmith; she is a researcher at a large institution. They have two small children. The wife describes herself as laboring to keep the relationship alive and to avoid separation. Biagio admits he has been behaving very selfishly lately, threatening to leave and being verbally violent with their children. He states that he no longer feels butterflies in his stomach; he feels claustrophobic and does not wish to take care of the three of them. As their therapist, I realize it would be even too easy to ally myself with the woman, very proactive, who labors for an honorable cause. It would be all too easy to criticize Biagio as all the people around them have already done. It would also be dangerous to confront Anna, who is under incredible stress about her responsibilities in the couple's dance. In the second session I decide to make a temporary alliance with the husband in order to understand what is taking place and to make his positioning comprehensible to Anna and myself. I need not collude with the process that has been taking place in recent months: Anna criticizing, pushing, and openly asking for more, feeling in the right to do so, and Biagio becoming more and more passive, feeling guilty. "Is there a common desire between the two of you?" I ask the couple, glancing at the man, trusting my therapeutic intuition and desiring to find a common ground after so much division they have spoken about. Immediately Anna is ready to answer; Biagio looks at me with eyes wide open, probably feeling trapped and overwhelmed by us women. He seems unable to say one word, and I feel he could run away. I interrupt Anna and ask Biagio if there have been other times in his life in which he felt exactly as he does now. I ask this with a tender voice and an inviting attitude, since I imagine him as a two-year-old child paralyzed with fear. He begins to cry and tells us that his father was a violent alcoholic who would always put him down and that it was dangerous to state his opinion; it was safer to hedge. Since he respects Anna a lot, he continues, he tries not to say what he really thinks, fearing he will hurt her. He therefore hides from her how he feels and does not open up. In a temporal ping-pong between past and present, we understand that Biagio is confused and frightened by his own feelings. He always thought that having a family was forever, since this was the way in which his violent father had been keeping them "prisoners". Now he has lost the desire to come home in the evening and this disturbs him greatly. He needs time. He does not consider Anna an enemy, and he hopes to be able to keep the family together. When we say goodbye at the end of the session, I say that it is clear that the common intent is keeping the family united and that we will try together to work in that direction.

I leave the session with the idea that we opened a new cognitive and emotional map and with a sense that we touched the depth of their feelings for each other. I reflect on my idea of a couple and of the difficulties of being in a relationship and my wish to learn from them.

Opening up to possibilities means to challenge the dominant discourse, go beyond the stability the system brings to us; it means to facilitate the creation of new possibilities, deconstruct ideas and habits, consider relationships and events from other points of view, open up to dreams and hypotheses that had no space before. It means to play, be ironic, be able to go against dominant traditions (Deleuze, 1983). The therapist, as co-author of the process, can propose, suggest, illuminate, deconstruct questions, never fully believing her theories. As Cecchin used to say, "Flirt with your hypotheses but never marry them".

The Depth of Our Fundamental Interchange

Self and other are at once knower and known, mutually entrenched in their special and unique encounter to try to make it become a collaborative performance. They exchange, collaborate, understand and misunderstand each other. After their encounter they become interdependent and influence each other, share an unconscious, the morphogenetic field of which Sheldrake (2011) speaks. The transformative inquiry is very much connected with this kind of creative encounter and with the co-created emotional path in which the algorithm of the heart plays a big part. We invite all the subjects in the room to participate in transformative experiences. The results of our interventions emerge from an interactive game in which the professional is not the only active subject.

Unintended consequences are the result of conjoint actions, not related specifically to one individual or the other, nor are they caused by external factors. Participants in interaction play an active role in tracing the path of the joint action, but the path itself is contingent, procedural and historical. In my opinion, it is useful to realize that we can only approach situations as they present themselves to us, without expecting to know a system "well" or "better". We should stop asking to know but rather ask to feel, to perturb, to make something happen in the here and now of the therapeutic context. Our knowing is always incomplete, observation always implies blind spots, we therefore cannot rely on top-down planning or only on what we understand. I am referring to the need that the clinician, abandoning the myth of control, is satisfied with provisional knowledge and works not to understand too soon and not to saturate her knowledge of the others – also that she trusts the self-healing capabilities of the system. I am speaking about an embodied transformative inquiry that emphasizes the circular interaction between the people involved in the here and now of a narrative. Here is an Ouroborean[7] alchemical image of the process: all the people involved should be curious about the nature of their meeting and about the outcomes they may co-create. New scripts become a cooperative co-production. Morphogenesis is the theme: how newness emerges, how order comes about from disorder and noise, how self-organization produces new organization (von Foerster), how the possible can actualize through the process of differences which does not mean diversity but rather intensity and individuation (Deleuze, 2003). Novelty is possible. The new is a singularity; it breaks a status quo, destabilizes the human becoming and the situation; it ruptures them. Differentiation is the process through which possibilities actually occur. It is the intensity of the encounter that leads to opening up to potentialities.

> People need to become poets and they become so through the questions from the clinician: it is important to ask questions that the individual has not thought of before. This offers the chance to step out of the usual blueprints, to invent new solutions.
>
> (Heinz von Foerster in an interview; Telfener, 1987, p. 43)

Mistakes

Within the systemic framework, it is a mistake to fear mistakes, since the possibility of a miscalculation is not separate from the possibility of understanding. Errors are important, and there is no logical way to avoid them in psychotherapy. Errors are signals that can help professionals to correct their process (they are usually within a behavioral domain). Keeney (1983) thinks that trying to avoid mistakes is a mistake since the basis for the self-correction emerges from the same possibility of generating errors and differences which allow us to change our behavior and the process. Therapists are always open to error because we carry the burdens of dominance, capitalism and colonialism too. Mistakes are signals; they are necessary in order to introduce differences that allow us to change our behavior and our premises. It is, however, a mistake not to realize that we have done something that is not working, that produces a homeostatic loop. Mistakes are inevitable. One day Anna telephoned me to say – to my surprise – that Biagio was a "bad narcissist". I did not stop her in time; I fell into the trap of the diagnosis. Then, realizing my mistake, I asked her to repeat her comment in the session in front of her husband. I told her I would not know how to deal with her "criticism" if it remained between us. She courageously revealed her "prejudice". I commented on the need to move from static descriptions to ongoing wishes and possibilities, and the process went on.

Impasse

Even impasse is an inevitable feedback of our ongoing process. It represents those situations in which we find ourselves all of a sudden without any hint. I am speaking of bifurcation points that we had not foreseen and that oblige us to take an alternative path. They derive from the story of the therapeutic process and of the encounter between client and therapist. They have to do with the clinical model and the context. They occur in space and time, signaling the necessity to think back the process; they can open up to significant evolutive moments.

More than once I felt I had reached an impasse with Biagio and Anna – when I felt that the process was stuck and that I had become bored or anxious, feeling a loss of energy and curiosity in the session; when Anna was coming in angry and discouraged and very critical, and all the process seemed influenced by negativity; when Biagio was more silent than ever, which made everybody lose hope for a breakthrough. Once I was in a personal difficult relational impasse with a friend who was very like Biagio, and this made me fearful of taking sides. Each time I decided that, instead of trying to change them or the situation, I would change my attitude towards them. In the session, I would try to organize a process that could become generative. I would use postcards or active role-playing between the two. I would co-create a sculpture or make them play a role reversal. I sometimes gave them feedback on my fantasies on how their rapport could evolve. My feelings have always been a good response to what they were bringing into the session and on how their relationship was proceeding: my boredom was the signal of a repetitive recursive pattern. My fear indicated that there was something neither they nor I was eager to deal with, a taboo that was not addressed and shared. My anger was the signal of a block in the process, the hypothesis that there was resistance.

Doctor Homeostat, Orthopedic Intervention

Lynn Hoffman used to warn her colleagues against becoming Doctor Homeostat, the professional who states the obvious and goes along with the self-regulation of the system not introducing news of difference. In order not to become like him, it is useful if we believe in the reciprocal relational process, if we understand its self-referencing,[8] if we perform operations upon operations.[9] We know that a therapist who is not able to imagine the evolutive forces and the resources that can be brought out becomes an anchor that holds the family blocked. Each time we intervene we can behave either in an orthopedic or in an evolutive mode. We can work for the *orthos*, the norm, or we can try to produce change. If we go with the description the system has brought to us, we risk remaining within the same frame: it becomes difficult to perturb since we accept already defined solutions, evident and simple.

Orthopedic interventions are those interventions that: endorse the explanation proposed by the clients; reduce complexity; apply universal categories; operate with the same premises as the system; remain trapped in the self-reference of the problem/solution; tend to normalize what is brought to the session, following society's prejudices and laws; create invisible collusions; place professionals in the position of Doctor Homeostat; tend to move the system into stable, unchanged behaviors. With Biagio and Anna, it would be orthopedic to strive to keep them together for the sake of their marriage and two small children. It would also be orthopedic to make an alliance with the woman to keep the family united. Even the choice of splitting the couple and working with the more energetic (Anna) would result in a catch that would further amplify the differences between the two. Falling into the trap of believing – as many women do – that in these hypermodern times (Telfener, 2018) men behave deficiently and are incapable of being nurturing in a relationship would have become a push towards the dominant social point of view. The remedy is trying to keep a balance, to feel sympathetic towards Anna and support her without criticizing Biagio. The remedy is to try to phantasize new options, in order not to block the system, to shift alliances, to look for resilience in both, to believe that they are trying and that some solution is at hand.

Our Inevitable Blindness

In addition to the freedom to trust intuition, to feel good in situations that are not under our control, and to trust others, allowing them to become our best collaborators, what does it mean to consider oneself blind? To be aware of the possibility of our blindness pushes us to trust in the order that derives from disorder and to trust the system's ability to self-heal. It requires us to take responsibility for the process and for the different layers that define concepts and information. The helping professional relationship asks for a high degree of reflexivity (that is the message of this whole chapter), otherwise the relationship becomes one of friendship. The risk of undesired outcomes emerges from this failure to consider therapy as a second-order process. The aim in therapy is not to fight the other's ideas and propositions, nor to arm wrestle, but rather to create a synergy. We might think of windsurfing, where we ride the waves, go where the wind takes us, proceed where it is possible, considering the wind, the tide, the waves and the sea currents, the surf we are surfing on, the sail, the keel, our muscles and our expertise. We go where the context of all the forces in which we are immersed takes us. We collaborate with our clients: we perturb, protect, challenge, defend, inspire, propose, suggest, feel; we introduce doubts and create provisional truths; we also confirm and highlight hypotheses and life scripts. Multiplicity creates its possibilities which emerge from the flux of what happens. We also risk resonating, colluding, participating in the creation of consensus and chronicity, we are in danger of burning out as professionals, to participate in a process that gets worse. The therapeutic process has to become reflexive so that the setting becomes an expressive one and the relationship one of collaboration. The example that comes to mind is a fish that swims in water while water is also inside it.

Collusion

Collusion has two faces. It is a useful step in the process of collaboration (a couple's collusion helps their marriage to continue) but is a dangerous interpersonal attitude in psychiatry. Collusion on a diagnosis prevents the introduction of new hypotheses, creating a status quo. It is a homeostatic trap unless we are aware of it. It is inevitable; it occurs in any given process since nowadays we live in a collusive culture (Telfener, 2018). In the phase of joining with a new system, it is a useful procedure to help understand how the system functions, by what rules it is governed, what emotions reign in it. To collude means to connect to a system (Laing, 1961), to make a structural coupling with it; it refers to the possibility of being temporarily incorporated into the system, of contributing to the equilibrium the system has established: the need to be reciprocally confirmed, as in falling in love, which Laing defines as "reciprocal shared deceit", in which each partner agrees to play the other's game, starting up a reciprocal confirming process.

Collusion has yet another meaning. It states the risk of continuing to think as the system does, the risk of falling into the field we have built together, of resonating with the usual praxis. In this case it means to lose the multidimensionality of the process, to adapt to an established and a priori definition, to photograph a reality locked in time and space, to be able to see only certain aspects of a complex reality, to set up actions/feelings that reify the status quo. Every clinician has to work on many planes. She connects what is happening here and now with what has already happened or may yet happen, with what she thinks about the situation, and with her past experience with other clients. When colluding, the professional loses the evolutive force, she falls into reifying the problem, not considering an evolutionary stance; she obeys the quest, considering only the observed system and leaving herself out of the picture, leaving contextual clues out of the process, often leaving time out. Colluding means obeying the mainstream, reifying a power relationship, falling into procedures, losing curiosity, "buying" the hypothesis of the working-net (enlarged system), responding to an emergency frame. It always implies not distinguishing between first- and second-order interventions. Handling collusion becomes vital for the professional to regain her potential to perturb. How can we try not to collude? By requiring people to distance themselves from their usual script; deconstructing the organization of the world as it is offered to us; encouraging irreverence in the interpretation of events (Cecchin et al., 1992).

I supervise a junior therapist who brings me a "difficult situation" in which she "feels stuck". The client, a 23-year-old woman, whom she sees once a week in individual sessions, cuts herself, eats very irregularly, is clearly underweight, and has a co-dependency relationship with a young man her age with whom she lives. The therapist has formed a good alliance. The client arrives on time; she seems moderately interested, passively participates in the process with a great deal of criticism of her family and the rest of the world. In the therapeutic processes some evolution seems to have taken place: she has left the verbally abusing boyfriend only to become promiscuous and has told her distant parents that she has been vomiting. By the time the therapist asks for supervision, both therapist and client had come to feel stuck and unhappy.

In our encounter, I realize that the psychologist has "bought" the woman's point of view: she too hates the client's father, whom she describes as stingy and uncaring, and disapproves totally of the mother, whom she describes as cold as an iceberg and critical. Like her client, the therapist sees no solution and opposes any hypothesis that enlarges the picture or suggests alternative narratives. The therapist has not realized that, having bought the client's premises, she is no longer able to introduce differences and to perturb the narratives they share. She has lost her curiosity, she has "married" the client's premises, and the two women go along in a mirroring process in which they both complain of the client's misfortune. The supervisor too needs to consider her own premises and decide which connections could be useful, without criticizing the professional, as the therapeutic system criticizes the parents and significant others in the picture (*fractal effect*, which is unavoidable[10]).

Resonance

Resonance is the movement and sound of many pairs of feet marching over a bridge; marching to one rhythm, they produce a single sound. In the same way, emotions become one when we are so involved in a narrative that we resonate with it, losing our sight and our perturbative force. Elkaïm (2008) proposed the theme of resonance as a situation in which the discourse is too close to us (delicate, sensitive, taboo, emotional, embedded). He would argue that when the clinician finds herself in the codified context of an encounter, the very first sentiment to emerge is bound not only to the person in front of her and to the implicit interlocutors – the colleagues, customers, clients, significant others – but to the professional herself, although it cannot merely be termed her personal feelings. The emotions and feelings that emerge have to do with the newly formed system and at the same time are related to the personal life of each of the people involved. These useful and disturbing emotions can indicate an important rule of the system of which we clinicians are now a part; the experience can offer a chance to understand what is going on in this new context. The analysis of our own feelings and sensations in the session lead to the discovery of a bridge that links us to the others at the precise moment when the process is taking place.

The resonance that emerges between professional and client is not just linked to the personal history of the interviewer or just to the members of that system. These common elements also concern other systems in the picture, such as the context in which a family has grown up, the supervision group the clinician participates in, and others. Transversally, resonance involves many interconnected systems in which we can find the same rule reproduced over and over. Resonance has an adaptive quality and a homeostatic one; I am emphasizing both. It is often inevitable. When it blocks the process, it may be overcome by teamwork, co-supervision, or reflection, by assumption of multiple stances or by awareness that it can occur.

In supervision I discovered that the therapist had a very contrarian attitude towards her own parents, whom she considered had been very neglectful while she was growing up. She told me she had worked in her own therapy on this specific aspect and believed she had resolved it. She was surprised by the questions about her childhood and late adolescence that were asked in supervision and immediately saw what she had not been seeing: she had resonated with her client's script, had identified with the story told, and had reified it. In this way she was keeping the plot alive and losing her perturbative force. She herself had suffered from neglect and had not yet overcome it, despite thinking otherwise, and she had concentrated far too long on her client's rage. When dealing with themes that are "too" close to us, we tend either to ignore them or to give them excessive emphasis. We can also transport ourselves and others into the realms of creativity and actions from which we return full of resources.

Chronicity

Every one of us has had to shoulder the responsibility of intervening in tough situations, with the task of deconstructing symptoms/problems and helping people to gain a new status. I would bet that each and every one of us professionals has at some point fallen into the trap of pathology and has been frightened by the sheer severity of the symptoms, has been caught in official nosology, has suffered from the disorientation it involves. We need time to learn that people are not their symptoms, that individuals and situations are constantly changing. The professional should take great care to help the evolutive process to begin again, certainly not taking the individual by the hand or pushing for change. It is in these cases that the self-regulatory abilities of organisms and institutions become interesting to monitor and never to forget.

"Competency is within people", says Eia Asen, "and our task is that of creating contexts where it becomes possible to make competency emerge" (Asen and Sholz, 2010). This positioning involves the need to look for and use all resources available (in the system, in the social setting of the clients, and in the therapeutic setting). We need to become witnesses to the potentials of both the individual and the system, and we need to imagine virtuous circles that emerge from the dance we perform together, accepting both problems and pains. The Milan school is famous for its faith in the capacities of its clients (as much as in its students) and in general of the "human becomings" to adapt and evolve. This faith also implies confidence in the perturbing capacities of the clinicians,[11] in the evolution of the context and in the possibility of utilizing the relationship as a primary tool in our work. The chronicizing process is often favored by collusion between the person asking for help and the person offering it, and even more frequently by collusion among all the professionals dealing with the same case. It is a consequence of the loss of a common project around a symptomatic occurrence. If institutions tend to work under pressure, if professionals fall into the trap of believing in pathology, if procedures become more important/urgent than people, clinicians lose their perturbative influence.

If a client gets worse, does it always make sense to double the number of sessions? To those reporting a worsening of their condition after a session, Gianfranco Cecchin used to propose a longer interval between sessions. "If you feel worse after a session, it could mean that the encounters are too perturbing and we need to increase the gap between sessions", he would say to the client. The relational meaning of this move is quite clear: avoid slipping into the logic of pathology; continue having faith in the person and their capacity to cope with even greater anxiety; do not allow symptoms to be used for blackmail; do not accept proxy. Exploit the vibrating quality of the region of intensities one is in "whose development avoids any orientation toward a culmination point or external end" (Deleuze and Guattari, 1987, p. 24).

Antonio, a young man of 20, was hospitalized after an automobile accident and a subsequent big fight with his father because he was confused, hyperactive and at risk of violence towards himself and others. A ward is a place where professionals share the same diagnosis, believe in medication and often think that if a crisis occurs around the age of 20, we need to speak of "psychosis". Antonio was treated as a sick person who needed to be contained through medication. The medication was "strong", and my client "woke up" (his word) three years later, fat, self-indulgent, having lost a piece of his life. His father had accepted the diagnosis and thought of him as an impaired person who would always need surveillance and help. His mother still wanted to fight for her son's well-being and asked for consultation. The three of them came to my office. Antonio, by then 24, was much appeased by medication. He acted like an eight-year-old boy asking for his mother's help. He would go grocery shopping with her and would watch television with her, holding hands. I analyzed the request when they were all together, then again when Antonio remained alone with me. When alone, he stated his desire to die, since his life meant nothing to him. I agreed that his life was worthless, and we made a deal: I would contact the hospital professionals in order to lower his medication and see if this would awaken him to life. We would decide his destiny only then, in six months' time, when the quality of his life was better.

After obtaining consent from Antonio's mother and the dubious agreement of his father, I needed to speak with the psychiatrist who had referred the parents to me. We spoke by telephone, and he declared he could not reduce the medication since Antonio could become very provocative and violent. I found myself in a paradoxical space where I could not operate: I could do nothing with the situation as it was. I therefore declared I would refuse to start therapy and would dismiss their request. I informed the family and excused myself. Two weeks later, the same psychiatrist, a professional I respect greatly, called and told me he would agree to my request until the first crisis, at which point he would resume medication. I could not accept this offer either, because the homeostatic forces in the system had been active for a long time and I could not assure either him or myself that there were not going to be any relapses. We ended the call at the same point: nothing was planned for Antonio's future.

After another two weeks, I received a call from Antonio's mother: the hospital had begun to reduce the medication and insisted he have therapy. Could I begin? No. I was very sorry, but I needed to speak with the psychiatrist since he was the professional in charge and I could not bypass him. We needed to agree not to work against one another instead of replicating the dynamics between mother and father, who never agreed. The next time we spoke, the psychiatrist acted softer: what about one year's time and me dealing with the possible crisis if it occurred? I accepted, telling him I would need his help, but we would act in agreement, keeping each other constantly up to date on what was happening. Therapy could begin.

I met with the whole family three times then decided to work with Antonio alone, since he needed to separate from his family of origin, and I did not feel comfortable to deal with the negative forces of the family as a whole. Their common history was one of sabotaging any change. The more the medication was abandoned, the better Antonio's spirits. He was quick and witty, and life was getting into our sessions and into his existence. We would surf the web, listen to music together, review his life through postcards. We would try to explain what had happened and look for the coherence of his story within the larger system. I kept an attitude of active research; I felt we were two scientists working on the same project, to understand what had happened and not let it happen again. Lightness was our mantra.

Clinical occurrences are at risk of chronicity when professionals fall into the trap of pathology, believing the dangers of symptoms and problems; when they lack coordination among themselves; enter into resonance and continue producing similar pathologizing dynamics; do not utilize a case manager who coordinates interventions and keeps in mind what has been happening and what has been done; work in institutions where the organization is based on a lack of a shared project; ignore health promotion and rehabilitation as possibilities within the institution's care. This risk is not due to the gravity of the situation itself but rather to how processes are dealt with. In order to avoid chronicity, it is necessary to shift from an intervention considered as a technique to one that makes processes and common meanings emerge from the problem-determined context.

The Risk of Iatrogenic Risk

Since therapists usually believe that people are always evolving and are capable of adapting, our objective is not to block their natural evolution. We need to be careful about how the interventions we propose may block/stabilize a process or make it generative. The therapeutic process can harm instead of healing. Such iatrogenic reactions are unintended consequences that emerge from interactive processes even when the model is correctly applied. They suggest that the worsening is not connected with the personality of the client or the difficulty of the situation but is caused by the relational dance performed in the therapeutic encounter. It is a phase, a harmful happening, a vicious circle that implies an increase in anxiety for the client, a sense of loss of self, of being transparent, thoughts of incapacity and inadequacy, a sense of chronic distrust in one's own judgment.

Literature on this subject is scarce. What little there is usually stresses multiple elements having to do with intrinsic characteristics. I prefer to emphasize those that deal with the summing up of the relations among the people involved: the therapist who turns on autopilot and performs stereotyped interventions, always the same; how the encounter is conducted; one's positioning in it; people made passive and who feel incompetent after too many interventions; medications that keep one's energy too low; offering many techniques without a frame that gives sense to them.

Here is an example:

Giovanna is a 41-year-old translator who has travelled and worked in many contexts both in Italy and abroad. She has been very competent and has had many recognitions in her career. After being left by her fiancé when she was 38 – after three years of living together – she had a breakdown and sought help and medication. The professional who saw her gave her antidepressants, which immediately made her feel "strange, like in an aquarium, as if between me and reality there were masses of dust and of distance". She describes her feelings to him, who suggests that she should continue the medication and wait for it to take effect. She returns two weeks later saying she feels more depressed than ever. She feels sluggish, as though something were slowing her down. She is afraid of this state because she has always tended to be a "doer", energetic and vigorous. The professional, seemingly identified with the symptoms, insists that she continue both her treatment and therapy with him. Giovanna will find herself one month later hospitalized in a hospital ward after attempting suicide. She had taken a full box of "her" pills, but called for help one hour later.

I intervene on behalf of Giovanna who asks for a consultation, feeling that her therapist was too critical toward her and indirectly accused her for being sneaky and not straight in the expression of her feelings. "I felt he thought of me as very sick and unaware", she tells me. I find myself sitting with a very scared and insecure lady, pleasant but showing neglect in her clothing: she would never have thought she could do anything so extreme, harming her life and actively intervening against existence. She has spent her last two months at home, alone, and has refused every job offer she has received lately. She feels confused and insecure and does not recognize herself. She has a sense of distrust in her own self-assessment and judgment. I have the feeling that the first thing to do is to deconstruct her sense of un-worthiness, to find an explanation for what happened, and to help her regain the image of herself she seems to have lost. We take into consideration the possibility that the medication had kept her energy lower than usual and that she had not recognized herself. She had therefore entered a clinging and insecure phase in which she had questioned her whole life. We hypothesize that these black holes are very uncomfortable but useful because one comes out of them feeling stronger and more aware. Giovanna's request is to go back to her usual self and to regain her strength and her competency. We will work on these terms in order for her to take a trip to Paris with regained confidence.

We need to inquire what interactional patterns have emerged and are maintained in the worsening process.

The concept of iatrogenic reactions should be part of the theoretical background of every clinician since only lucid awareness and critical distance can help professionals not to fixate on a single interpretation of what is happening or to follow a line of intervention that is more consistent with who the clinician is than with the client's seeking health. To be mistaken in psychotherapy is possible, at times inevitable, but to persist is always destructive. Malpractice is the worsening of a iatrogenic emotion. It happens in those cases in which the clinician persists with no awareness of her involvement in the process.

How to Deal with Transformation: Responsibility as Political, Ethical, and Aesthetic Stances

"Every time I act in the here and now", von Foerster states at a conference on ethics (1990), "not only do I change, the Universe changes as well. This positioning inexorably ties the subject and its actions with everybody else, it establishes a prerequisite to found an ethics". Within this interdependence between the subject and the universe, the professional will not only be able to enjoy the multitude of connections she will experience. She will also form webs of ecologies and be involved in the choices that the explanations contain. She must be considered accountable for what happens in the encounters, as she is socially defined as the one who has a public role and is paid for her work as a family and community therapist (Telfener, 2011).

I think of therapy as the harmonization of musical instruments that need to find a common rhythm in order to synchronize and allow differences to emerge. A sort of reciprocal regulation takes place in all systemic work in order to create together an assemblage of voices and bodies. What does it mean to synchronize, to harmonize, to promote evolution? It means to give space to what can happen, to tolerate chance, possibilities, imagination and love. To manage vitality and style, which is how to approach Otherness. To be available to transform our ideas and presuppositions by changing the way we observe, describe, feel and participate in the observing system. We must act differently in order to know differently.

We therefore perform political and poetic acts. The first has to do with the fact that we are moving beyond objectifications, intervening all the time, respecting the singularity of the encounter, freeing life, liberating potentials. We are maximizing connections. The poetic space is run by the co-construction of meaningful distinctions that make a difference and make people come together. As Marcelo Pakman proposes (Pakman, 2018), poetics is a constructionistic practice that does not look for meanings in irrational behaviors but rather declares that all behaviors are socially acceptable, factual, and open to meaningful interpretations. The poetics approach allows one to move between different interpretative frames, sharing more than one positioning at the same time, focalizing on making explicit and clear the mechanism that makes the proposals acceptable, effective and meaningful.

From a constructive point of view, ethics is an integral part of any action we take. The ethical stance is assumed by any professional through the responsible choices she subjectively makes, because we need constantly to decide regarding decisions that are in principle undecidable. It becomes essential to ask oneself how to make a therapeutic reality emerge in which it is possible to intervene; how not to become Doctor Homeostat; how not to risk the risk of iatrogenic risk (a second-order operation); how not to collude with the system or with the individual; how to work without imposing one's values. A good question we can ask ourselves could be: "How am I participating in perpetuating the symptom and maintaining the premises that organized it?", "In what way is the process that I have collaborated to create evolutionary or homeostatic?"

Responsibility concerns patterns that either favor or hinder the creation of shared events and the emergence of an evolutionary reality. Within the frame of construction, we are given back the freedom to define each happening and to choose the best way of participating in any ensuing problematic event. The meaning of what a clinician does is negotiated through an interactive embodied process in which all the participants are co-authors. Ethics becomes an implicit attitude expressed through responsibility, which is imperatively explicit. Aesthetic is the "tension between diversity and coherence: the coexistence of multiplicity and unity, difference and repetition", as Maria Esther said in a conference where we were together (2019).

Responsibility for responsibility refers to having to account, first of all, to oneself for the process of co-constructing social realities that are realized in the interaction.

What I have put on paper is the result of my life path. It also results from my awareness of living in a constantly evolving, breathing universe where every element does its best. Creation is extreme: it needs strength, time, many actors and so much difference. We live in an undetermined world in which we cannot have a linear, plain influence. The creative evolution involves every human being, even more so us health professionals who perform the task of amplifying processes and help to get out of situations of stress, malaise and illness. As systemic professionals, we are "between" mind and heart, social and individual, intra-psychic and relational, unconscious and principles of reality. I will end with two gifts to the reader. One is the ethical imperative my teacher Heinz von Foerster insisted on: "Act always in order to enhance the number of choices for yourself and for others". The second gift is a word in the Zulu language of South Africa. It is *sawubona*, which means, "I see you and by seeing you I bring you into being". We could add, "I bring you and myself into being".

Notes

1 The clinician will be described as "she" since the author is female.
2 I will often use the word "dance" which can be compared to a dialogue, written, spoken, felt, acted with another person who allows me to tune in with him/her, after which I know something more than before. Knowing according to systemic epistemology builds itself as action.
3 The observer is embedded in the observations s/he makes, which are not absolute but always relevant to her/his systems of coordinates.

4 Lines of flight can be enhanced by the encounter with the professional, introducing disorder to create new order.
5 Lethe in Greek mythology is the river of oblivion.
6 According to von Foerster, it is only those questions that are in principle undecidable that we can answer. The moment we have the freedom to make a choice, we immediately have the responsibility for our answer. This means to take an ethical stance.
7 The archetypal snake swallows its own tail, giving birth to what comes after, in a full immersion with the process of creation.
8 I am speaking of a recursive process: the Jorge Luis Borges story of Shahrazad comes to mind. The princess tells the story of her life and starts from scratch each time she arrives at a certain passage.
9 How not to fall into homeostasis: consider the possibility of blind spots; do not understand too fast; know temporarily; allow for unsaturated narratives; give support to evolutive potentialities; break the psychological coherence with which people come in, the self-reference which includes the problem/symptom.
10 A fractal is an image that is always the same even at different levels of sameness. A cauliflower has a fractal shape: each floret has the same shape, which is in turn the same as the whole; a pine tree is similar. I am using this image to propose how often in many processes this sameness comes about: the process that takes place in the client's family has been reproduced in the sessions. The supervisor must be careful not to reproduce the same critical process.
11 It is important that the clinician has confidence in her perturbative capacities and in the evolutive force of each encounter.

References

Asen, E. and Sholz, M. (2010). *Multi-Family Therapy, Concepts and Techniques.* Abingdon: Routledge.

Bianciardi, M. and Telfener, U. (2014). *Ricorsività in psicoterapia.* Turin: Bollati Boringhieri.

Cavagnis, M.E. (2019). *The Visible and the Invisible, Boardering Change in Systemic Family Therapy.* Presentation at the conference EFTA-SIPPR. Naples, September 11–14.

Cecchin, G., Lane, G. and Ray, W. (1992). *Irreverence: A Strategy for Therapists' Survival.* London: Karnac.

Deleuze, G. (1983). *Che cos'è l'atto di creazione?* Naples: Cronopio edizioni.

Deleuze, G. (2003). *Difference and Repetition.* Edinburgh: Edinburgh University Press.

Deleuze, G. and Guattari, F. (1983). *Anti-Oedipus: Capitalism and Schizophrenia.* Minneapolis, MN: University of Minnesota Press.

Deleuze, G. and Guattari, F. (1987). *A Thousand Plateaus: Capitalism and Schizophrenia.* Minneapolis, MN: University of Minnesota Press.

Elkaïm, M. (2008). The use of resonance in supervision and training. *Human Systems,* 19(1), 16–25.

Hoffman, L. (2012). The art of "withness": A new bright edge. www.systemics.eu/the-art-of-withness-a-new-bright-edge-lynn-hoffman/

Keeney, B.P. (1983). *Aesthetics of Change.* New York: The Guilford Press.

Kinman, C. (2017). The thing in the bushes: From commodities to ecologies. *Human Systems,* 28(2–3), 199–234.

Laing, R.D. (1961). *The Self and Others: Further Studies on Sanity and Madness.* London: Tavistock.

Pakman, M. (2018). *Immagine e immaginazione in psicoterapia: al di là della scienza empirica e della svolta linguistica.* Rome: Alpes.

Sheldrake, R. (2011). *The Presence of the Past: Morphic Resonance and the Habits of Nature.* London: Icon Books.

Telfener, U. (1987). Heinz von Foerster: Costruttivismo e psicoterapia. In M. Ceruti and U. Telfener (eds), *Sistemi che osservano.* Rome: Astrolabio.

Telfener, U. (2011). *Apprendere i contesti.* Milan: Cortina.

Telfener, U. (2018). *Letti sfatti, l'amore in epoca ipermoderna.* Florence: Giunti.

von Foerster, H. (1984). *Observing Systems.* Seaside, CA: Intersystems.

von Foerster, H. (1990). Ethics and second order cybernetics. Plenary session at the conference Systémes, Etique, Perspectives en Thérapie Familiale. Paris, 4–6 October.

von Foerster, H. (1992). Letologia vis à vis con gli indeterminabili, indecidibili, inconoscibili. In P. Perticari (ed.), *Conoscenza come educazione.* Milan: Angeli.

Chapter 6

Aesthetics, Ethics and Politics in Childhood Matters

Maria Esther Cavagnis and Inga-Britt Krause

Introduction

Our clinical work with children offers a very special and extraordinary opportunity to notice and take account of both the inside of relationships and the dynamic of systemic processes. In this chapter we explore this in terms of what work with children and families can contribute to the ethics and aesthetics in systemic practice. As described by Maria Esther in Chapter 3, in working with children and in mapping the therapeutic space, we are creating a new social landscape that makes momentary dispositions which drag us into new territories and possibilities. This is what Deleuze and Guattari call "lines of flight" (Deleuze and Guattari, 2013 (2008)).[1] "Lines of flight" refer to the opportunities which escape naming and endless mechanisms of capture and suffocation, and which therefore may transform our existence. This offers other possibilities different from the readings of the genogram, which to some extent relies on the conjecture of the past. We do not want to claim that the past is irrelevant for the relationships between children and their carers. This would be to discount and ignore a whole body of anthropological and other work on kinship and relationships between genders. Rather we see the past as relevant insofar as the experiences of the past are organizing for the present and mapping them makes it possible to find new modes of organization. Nor do we ignore the work of developmental psychology or psychoanalysis. This body of work has not only been important to the thinking of Deleuze and Guattari, and Bateson, it has also offered possibilities for systemic psychotherapists to rethink the way families are systems and in particular to take into account the multiple positions available to any one person in them and therefore providing an avenue of access to the dynamic processes inside and outside relationships. Our ideas attempt to move towards a theory, which avoids being cast in a particular political and ideological straightjacket. In this chapter we suggest first, that systemic psychotherapists, child psychotherapists and other child professionals have approached childhood without taking proper account of *difference*, in effect considering childhood and child development to take one path, namely that of Western capitalist

DOI: 10.4324/9780429437410-6

societies. Second, we critique the ideological aspects of psychology in which generalization and universalization have annulled the unique aspects of life as irrelevant or pathological. Along with this, systemic psychotherapy has also tended to ignore the invigorating and revolutionary aspects of childhood as well as the dynamic potential in any relationship or collection of relationships. In other words, we claim that insofar as finding spaces in our systemic psychotherapeutic work where experimentation, discovery and creativity can grow, our work with children is a promising area to examine and develop.

We are two women from different cultural backgrounds who for different reasons have been disenchanted with the current state of thinking and practice in systemic psychotherapy. Maria Esther is a child psychotherapist who became a family therapist as she was drawn to open broader contexts in her practice with children in order to understand non-individual ways of living and relating, which could expand intra-psychic explanations. Britt is a social anthropologist and a systemic psychotherapist who early in her career read *Naven* and who since then has been intrigued about the relationship between social science and psychotherapy. We are both mothers, but our children have grown up with different conventions and we ourselves are aware of differences between us. For one thing we do not speak the same language. However, although we do not share a common first language, we have found we do share a sense of understanding of the task of systemic psychotherapy. Although coming from psychology and anthropology respectively we both think about ontology as a process of constant differentiation, and believe it impossible to separate the psyche from what is social and cultural. Moreover, we regard those processes as being deeply implicated in the production of subjectivity (Cavagnis, 2014; Krause, 2012).

We consider that with the fall of modernity everything is in doubt and our systemic theories cannot help us much, since they cannot be separated from the analytical-political keys of which they are part and therefore the theories themselves are the effect of an evolutionary, Eurocentric and phono-phallus centrist epistemology. These issues cannot be avoided by clinicians, and in particular clinicians who practice with children. The central question is this: how do we think about the processes of subjectivation? How do we think about what happens with a child, with his/her existence from the beginning and during the process of living? Does he/she evolve? Is the process structured? What remains and what changes? What makes someone recognize him or herself as being him or herself and keeping certain ways of living, which may generate misery or unhappiness? These questions are the questions of the clinic, of philosophy and of the social sciences, which we want to see as heterogeneously connected together problematizing the complex field of "subjectivity". Binaries, which in the past defined different positions, such as innate/acquired; individual/social; nature/culture; interiority/exteriority cease to be options for thinking about subjectivity. We can only study how this modern-colonial subjectivity has been constituted and how it can be deconstructed. The psychology of development poses certain evolutionary, ascending hierarchical modes just as psychoanalysis proposes universal modes, centered on the Oedipus triangle, as an approach to think about the development of a psychic apparatus and its structures. The revolution of systemic thinking consisted precisely in focusing on the relationship between phenomena and the specific contexts in which they happen. From the discoveries of quantum physics onwards, we have learnt that objects, which were once thought of as elementary units existing before, implied that the idea of organization had lost ground vis-à-vis that of totality. Instead, with Elkaïm we conceptualize system as an emergence of interrelationships, which are organizing and become organized, that is any interrelation endowed with a certain stability or regularity takes on an organizational nature and becomes a system (Elkaïm, 1990; Morin, 1990; Pakman, 1994). The organization is the relationships of relationships, it produces its elements and its edges and at the same time maintains the system. The discourse of modernity has turned what is a verb (a process, namely organizational activity) into a noun (the organization). This idea of self-organization is restated by Deleuze and Guattari (Deleuze and Guattari, 2013 (2002)) and refers to the core of Bateson's work and systemic thinking.

In this chapter we begin by examining Deleuze's ideas with respect to children, a crucial aspect of his thinking about those questions, which we posed above about how to understand "the subject" and the process of subjectivization and how we work clinically with children. Deleuze himself commented on the work of Melanie Klein in several passages (Deleuze and Guattari, 2004 (1980)) and we will briefly summarize how we understand this debate in relation to the practice of systemic psychotherapy. In light of this we then move on to discuss child development and attachment. Here a cross-cultural perspective is particularly useful as a position from which to critique Eurocentric theories, which propagate universal modes of understanding centered on certain types of family organization and emotional outlooks. We suggest that the narrowness of thinking about childhood in systemic psychotherapy has contributed to systemic psychotherapists being ill equipped to imagine ways of childrearing and child development which do not fit with a Western capitalist outlook and temperament. We do not think it essential to have a general theory of child development. However, we do think that a therapist needs to have an idea about how she thinks about the processes of the production of subjectivity and that this implicates a set of interconnected themes around the processes of childhood, culture, subjectivity and intersubjectivity. We then move on to consider the development of genograms as a way of depicting family relationships, contributing to an unhelpfully static picture of families and relationships. We offer the complementary approach of cartography and comment on the differences between these two ideas. We further suggest that genograms limit the creativity of psychotherapists as well as the possibility of mapping. When a genogram is drawn, the field of the thinkable is limited. Genograms offer a single determined way of considering relationships and relating, a reading, which easily becomes totalizing. We will offer examples from our own clinical practice. We finish the chapter with a general discussion. Rather than focusing on what to represent, we suggest that the work needs to focus on the experiencing of being present in different paths. In general then, in this chapter we hope to alert systemic psychotherapists to the most important points made by Deleuze and Guattari with respect to children, which we consider offer the possibility for breaking free from dominant assumptions in psychotherapeutic work with children and families and hence for systemic psychotherapists to become more creative about the potential multiplicities inside all relationships. Rather than limit our work to the personal and the possessive in the sense of "my life is my world", we suggest, together with other authors, that relationships are not with total people or objects, but unique ways of relating through partiality and multiplicity.

Systemic Psychotherapy and Deleuze's Children

It is a frequently heard comment in systemic psychotherapy training contexts that, compared to our colleagues in child psychotherapy or child psychology, our trainees do not learn much about children or child development. Indeed, in the UK and Latin America, apart from those clinicians who work with children in the narrative tradition, there are only a small number of books addressing how to work systemically with children (Cavagnis, 2009; Vetere and Dowling, 2016; Wilson, 1998). Yet, systemic psychotherapists do of course meet with families, who consult about their children. How might we understand this apparent inconsistency? There has been a tendency for systemic psychotherapists to take a certain pride in offering a general view of relationships and relationships between relationships as systems, and in this way avoid directly thinking about the processes of history or development by focusing on the whole or the totality rather than on the (often uneven and unpredictable) processes behind that totality. Looking back to the origin of systemic ideas, or rather as these ideas have been put into practice since the arrival of systemic psychotherapy, we find that much can be said about the background and the context of systemic psychotherapeutic work with children, and both the contributions and limits these views have provided for our own work.

The general theory of open systems maintains that the tendency of the system is to unify in its different forms: homeostasis-equifinality-totality (Bertalanffy, 1969 (1976); Watzlawick and Beavis, 1997 (1991)). So how is a change possible? Traditionally, there seems to have been two possible alternatives: reproduction of the totality or the destruction of the system (Prigogine, 1983). The systemic principle of totality holds that everything is related to everything else, so that a change in one part affects the whole. This is a functionalist theory as understood in the tradition of Durkheim, Talcott Parsons and Radcliffe Brown.[2] The subject seems to participate in a relational game that catches him or her in a plot whose density makes his individuation more or less difficult. To think of the system as a whole or as a unity implies a structure and an organization that can only tolerate a finite quantum of possible changes (Thom, 1977). Recall the principle of equifinality and the threat that organizational change implies for a system. This conceptualization is linked to the idea of structure, in which relations are dependent and internal to the terms. There is no independence, there is no possible autonomy of the terms since the elements contain in themselves the structure of the whole. The parties are co-involved or co-involving and their continuity and cohesion are assured by the whole. The parties refer to the whole since the only possible actions they can undertake are in relation to the whole. This results in movement tending to go in one direction such as in evolution, an uninterrupted movement towards totality, rather than a facilitation of the possibility of indeterminacy. In the field of family therapy, structural models have argued that the functional structure must be maintained for the healthy emotional development of family members. This meant that the boundaries that differentiated one subsystem from another, the hierarchies between them etc., must be carefully guarded by therapists (Haley and Hoffman, 1968 (1967); Madanes, 1981 (1984); Minuchin, 1974 (2003); Watzlawick and Beavis, 1997 (1991)). Within this approach it is necessary to take care that the parents do not lose their place of authority, the limits of which establish adequate differentiation with the children, that they keep their agreements within the couple so as not to confuse the children with their differences etc. Even when a family member is missing such as in fostering and adoption, that function can be covered by designating the correct terminology to step and foster relationships and this being backed up by legal processes (Bourdieu, 1998). Many therapists (systemic and other) continue to practice according to these principles since these have been naturalized and institutionalized as universal and unquestionable truths: "A father is a father, a son is a son, and things should not be confused if we want a healthy society". In this universe of the one and where each thing is clearly different from the other, there is little place for the new.

This path is directed towards the progressive differentiation and autonomization of the "children", in the manner of cells that differentiate and then divide again and again to continue fulfilling the functions that allow us to stay alive. In first-order cybernetics it was argued that if this does not happen, the system is destroyed. Later with the theory of chaos and cybernetics of the second order, the option of bifurcation[3] was introduced. However, it is not clear how that mutation was considered possible. Where would those elements capable of assembling something different and new come from if each of them contains the information of all? Even in the conceptualization of complex systems by Edgard Morin (1990) his idea of totality is supported by the hologrammatic vision of the system. "The whole is in the part and the part is in the whole" (Morin, 1981). This refers to the idea that in the production of the whole the parts are related and in turn each part has the information of the whole, in the same way that any cell in our body contains the genetic information of the whole. We reiterate: from this perspective it is difficult to glimpse the production of the new, of the discontinuous, and of the unexpected.

As systemic psychotherapists we recognize this description of a system as well as the accompanying difficulties it articulates when it comes to thinking about change, the direction of change and difference. Yet we all know from our practice that it is the new, the discontinuous and the unexpected which frequently confronts us in our work. Deleuze and Guattari address these difficulties with the concept of "multiplicity". In this they build on the work of Freud and later Klein insofar as they discover the category of multiplicity in Freud's work (Deleuze and Guattari, 2004 (1980); Freud, 1918 (1976)) and its continuity in Klein's notion of partial objects (Klein, 1932 (1950)). Systemic psychotherapists are fond of distancing themselves from the psychoanalytic idea of the primacy of the "father" and the "mother". Yet, these ideas echo right through the discipline both in the development of first and second order outlined above, in the theory of life cycles and in systemic uses of maps generally referred to as genograms. We therefore also have much to learn from the assessment provided by Deleuze and Guattari of the ideas of Freud and Klein. We will address the issues of genograms separately below; here we focus on the notions of multiplicity and partiality.[4]

We may begin by acknowledging that things are related to each other in many different ways. There is no relationship that encloses them all, there is no being that contains everyone else. Deleuze explains this with respect to context, which he here refers to as a milieu:

> a milieu is made up of qualities, substances, powers and event: the street for example, with its materials (paving stones), its noises (the cries of merchants), its animals (harnessed horses) or its drama (a horse slips, a horse falls down, a horse is beaten...).The trajectory merges not only with the subjectivity of those who travel through it, but also with the subjectivity of the milieu itself, insofar as it is reflected in those who travel through it.
>
> (Deleuze, 1997, p. 61 (1996, p. 98))[5]

In these multiplicities there are discontinuities and consequently there is always something which escapes. What escapes is what the movement does, what it creates, what it innovates. It does not deny the processes of unification and composition, but recognizes the contingent given the innumerable possibilities. The idea of multiplicity does not deny the system, but proposes it as a tendency to unity constituted by a network of overlapping relationships without closure. They constitute partial connections and are conditions for the possibility of emergence of the new as a permanent becoming. The idea of multiplicity is linked to the idea of infinity. May explains this as follows:

> If we have a taste for paradox, which Deleuze does, we might say that the only being is the being of becoming... And that being is multiplicity, difference. It is not a multiplicity, that is a Many as opposed to a One. The One – duration, substance – is multiplicity itself. Multiplicity, difference, is not transcendent; it is immanent. Multiplicity is the affirmation of unity.
>
> (May, 2005, p. 60)

The key is to differentiate multiple (adjective linked to many of one) as when we say "there is a great multiplicity of types of insects" with multiplicity as a noun as Deleuze uses it where the number is a multiplicity (Bergson, 1960; Deleuze, 2014). Deleuze and Guattari take up the notion of partial objects, derived from the theories of Melanie Klein, by renaming them in the notion of desiring machines (later referred to as assemblages).[6] Machines are presented as a series of intensive multiplicities that are connected to each other in a rhizomatic way and distributed over the surface of the body[7] that resists being totalized or hierarchized. Deleuze questions the Kleinian theory of partial objects based on a strong criticism of the notion of totality. Klein's partial objects are causal mechanisms (such as in introjection and projection), which produce certain effects, which are good or bad. This, Deleuze suggests, is an idealist reading of partial objects (Deleuze and Guattari, 2004, p. 48) first because the Kleinian partial objects are considered to be "ghosts" (Fraiberg, 1975) and therefore not able to produce anything real, and second because again the schizo-paranoid object is considered pre-oedipal and thus refers back to a whole (Oedipus) from which nothing can escape. It all comes back to the Mother and the Father (Deleuze, 1994, pp. 130ff) and Klein cannot conceptualize these partial objects except in relation to whole persons, they cannot in themselves be desiring machines. In contrast, with desiring machines everything works at the same time, in a sum that never brings its parts together into a whole. There is instead an affirmation of multiplicity and emergence.

> A child does not play only mom/dad. He also plays the sorcerer, the cowboy, the police, the thief, the train and the cars. The train is not necessarily dad, nor the mom station. It is evident that the presence of parents is constant and that the child can do nothing without them. But this is not the problem. The problem lies in knowing if everything that concerns you is lived as a representative of the parents.
>
> (Deleuze and Guattari, 2004, p. 50)

We read these ideas as an invitation to resist the pressure and the temptation to look for the manifestly latent, to what we already "sort of" know in our work with families and children. We need to resist interpretation in terms which are already related to what we know about the past and in particular to past relationships with mothers and fathers. So for example in a therapy session with a Greek/Afro Caribbean mother and a mixed race daughter, both of whom had experienced much adversity and abuse, the six-year-old girl was making many drawings in each session. These drawings were all of multiple princesses, all of them white, with blond hair and long gowns flowing to the floor looking out at the viewer with smiles, stars and suns around their heads. In each drawing there was also a cat somewhere in the corner and in one drawing there was a much bigger cat with wings. There was much talk of the princesses about their sunny disposition and their beautiful hair and dresses and the contradiction between this, the color of the skin of the mother and the little girl and the past experience of both of them. There was talk about the girl cheering up her mother and coving over the difficulties with these sunny drawings. In all this talk the cats hardly got a mention. When the girl was asked about the cats with a slight expectation of something representing something else, she answered that she had just learnt to draw cats and that she was practicing this new skill! The question is, could the therapists refrain from interpreting this along familiar lines or could the cats point to something new?

In another example, Ivan a four-year-old Argentinian, middle class boy, was attending a therapy session in which both his parents were present. Different professionals had diagnosed Ivan with different disorders: one, an individual therapist, thought that he had OCD because Ivan did not like things being moved around; his teacher thought that Ivan was suffering from ADHD because he did not pay enough attention in his kindergarten; one psychiatrist diagnosed Oppositional Syndrome because Ivan did not accept the limits his parents set him and instead would run away and try to lock himself in his room. Ivan's parents were unhappy together and were both preoccupied, one with an impending operation and the other with work. In one of the sessions, while the parents talked about their concern and helplessness in setting boundaries, Ivan pretended to be writing, filling the blackboard with characters perfectly aligned in two columns (he can't write yet). He commented on his drawing "...this is the index of an encyclopedia on insects", and asked parents and therapist to choose which insects they wanted to learn about. They agreed to talk about butterflies. Initially, Ivan talked about the process of transformation from chrysalis to butterfly. The therapist made the assumption that Ivan had little parental support, and asked "Who helps her?" And the boy said: "Nobody, they do it alone". Then he said that spiders are a danger to the life of butterflies and the adults went back to their line of questioning: "...and who can help the butterfly?" Ivan said: "No one" and both the parents and the therapist continued "...and the butterfly's parents and family cannot help?" Ivan became visibly upset and said, "No, butterflies don't make families! Only animals make a family. Butterflies do not make anything, they only live with others, but they do not make anything".

Systemic psychotherapists may not feel so bound to an interpretation leading back to the mother and the father, or various representations of these relationships, but are we able to keep in mind multiplicity and emergence within the constraint and limitations of the consulting room and the institutionalized processes behind this setting? Are we able to consider the drawing of the cat as an event, which emerges as a differential burst of forces? When talking about an "event" we have to think of a multiplicity of forces. Events are characterized by the effects or the multiple senses they generate. Events are not preceded by causes that allow them to be anticipated before, but may result from minimal, banal or imperceptible situations. In this way we think not of a closed system of forces but of a dynamic of forces. This difference in intensive forces cannot be defined from an instance outside of it that is transcendent. An event manifests itself in a state of affairs, a singularity, that is to say in every event the moment of its realization is present (Deleuze, 1994). We are in a plane of immanence.[8]

Attachment and Child Development

We argue that the way we include and exclude the cultural aspects of our readings and the way we represent children in our societies are political actions with disciplinary effects. To appreciate this it is necessary to deconstruct the universalist and generalist discourses of developmental and educational psychology, as well as review studies about childhood. It is in line with this that we re-examine attachment theory in this chapter.

Along with a general lack of attention to children and child development in systemic psychotherapy has also come a lack of attention to attachment theory in traditional systemic training, at least in the UK. The exception to this has been the work of Byng-Hall, who wrote about attachment patterns in families and family scripts (Byng-Hall, 1995). Recently this has changed and attachment theory is now taught to systemic trainees as well as written about in general introductory books (Dallos and Draper, 2005) but without a concerted attempt to track the implications and contradictions this might pose for systemic thinking generally. In other psy-disciplines attachment has become an influential perspective on child development, child-rearing practices and clinical practice with one derivative, mentalization, receiving widespread attention (Fonagy et al., 2004). After centuries in which the image of "the natural" has been used to regulate the structures of society and parenting systems, particularly the position of women in relation to children, a legitimate skepticism has been generated regarding forms of research, which propose the co-production of biological aspects together with the social and political aspects. Family sociologists and anthropologists have placed attachment theory and evaluations of it as part of the discursive "software" that operates the "hardware" of bio-political surveillance and the discipline of child rearing overseen by the state (see for example LeVine, 2014; LeVine et al., 1996; Quinn and Mageo, 2013). From Oakley (1971) to Koffman (2015) feminist academics have also described the theorizations about attachment as expressing a conservative desire to hold women accountable for their mode of bringing up children, presenting this as an issue related to the future good of the nation. In a society in which women have the primary responsibility for the care of babies, babies also demand the availability of mothers, so that it appears that attachment processes themselves cause the baby to look for a discriminated attachment figure as the solution to their distress. All this appears to support conservative economic and political ideologies, which rely on the emergence of self-sufficient individuals as a natural process, which does not implicate health, social or political resources.

Guattari wrote that "an ethological perspective recognises that the child, as an individualised organic totality, constitutes an intersection between the multiple material biological, socioeconomic and semiotic components that cross it" (Guattari, 2015 (2013, p. 160)). The inclination of a baby to seek protection from their caregiver when alarmed is not a unilateral mechanism, but an assembly that is performed differently in different micro-social contexts and which in turn shapes them. In our perspective the individual is not prior to his/her environment, but is co-determined, constituted within and through the interaction of patterns of affections, movements and the changes of the bodies that occur in relationships. The implication in terms of how we should understand the "attachment system" is that the reality of that system, such as the classifications through which its variations are described, does not pre-exist in the contexts, processes and interaction through which it occurs. This implies that attachment theory has been used to affirm the affective value of the family at the expense of its associated environment. What is at stake is not so much what attachment is, but how it is being used. Here is an example in a statement from a television interview about a group of young people who committed criminal acts in Argentina:

> When children have not enjoyed a secure attachment, they have difficulty developing satisfactory emotional ties, they are usually violent, they have a bad relationship with authority figures, they do not conform to the rules and they have bad relationships with their parents. Later, as adults they often end up becoming troublemakers, and run the risk of falling into crime and drug addiction.
>
> (Rodriguez Muñoz, 2020)

This extract shows how the use of "attachment" can be a way to hide and oversimplify the heterogeneity of forces at play, between objects, and bodies implicated in fields as different as child behavior, crime, human genetics,

Otherness, law etc. This kind of use of "attachment" is worrying because it connotes attachment as a linear and unique causal predictor and explanation. We think that critical deconstruction work is necessary and one way to begin to do this is by looking at child development from the point of view of different cultural perspectives, but also from the perspectives of different inclinations and events in which we take part in the therapy room as suggested in the example of work with Marysol. Marysol was a ten-year-old Argentinian girl from an impoverished background. Marysol had grown up on the street in a small town in the interior of Argentina. Her mother, an alcoholic and perhaps mentally ill, had seven other children by different biological fathers. She raised her children in poverty, often resorting to begging and robbery. Marysol herself was a victim of sexual abuse since the age of six. She was given up for adoption twice and on both occasions the foster parents returned her to the authorities because of her misbehavior. The therapy session was part of a third attempt at adoption. This adoptive mother was a 40-year-old single woman, a social worker, a feminist, and a women's rights activist, who was very concerned and upset about Marysol's horrifying experiences and afraid of not being able to manage these for Marysol, and she sought therapeutic help in order to complete the adoption process in the best possible way. This new mother could not understand why, despite the change in her life situation, Marysol continued to take objects or money from other people when she was given everything she wanted or why Marisol constantly asked for more, stole, lied and climbed up on older men's knees asking for money. Marysol also showed violent, sexually inappropriate behavior to other children. The would-be adoptive mother's misery was intense and often somewhat unbearable, and the therapist (Maria Esther) was afraid that she might give up on adoption – it seemed Marysol also feared this. In a therapy session Marysol told the therapist and her adoptive mother that her biological mother demanded that she steal and that she was told she couldn't use the money to buy food, even if she was hungry. She and her brother sometimes used the money to buy food and then had to lie to avoid punishment. Marysol told the adults about those terrible experiences, one by one. An intense sadness fell upon us all in the therapy room. In this session while the mother recounted in anguish the events of the week, the girl began to play with her top, which had a sequined heart on the front that would change from black to silver as she slid her hand over it. Maria Esther took time to think about how to intervene and at the same time about how to control her own anxiety. She focused her attention on the figure on Marisol's top as Marisol played with it, and asked her to keep changing the color, to no other purpose than to gain control of her own feelings. Marysol did this fast, she rushed. Maria Esther asked her to do it more slowly, more gently, warning her she may tear the sequined heart. Marysol did as she was told and asked: "Why do you want me to do this?" And after a while, as Maria Esther started to feel that the game made sense, she, blushing with joy, said: "I understand! I understand!

Do you mean that the change takes time?" The mother joined in to say: "Of course, sometimes I am unaware that this is a process. She is learning to live differently". Playing with her top had enabled us to find a line of flight. We had played without a conscious purpose, and play thus became an expression of affect, intensities and forces that showed the way out of the situation and took us to other possible territories.

Children Here, There, and Everywhere

Bateson did not work specifically with young children, although as an anthropologist relationships between children and adults (carers) were of course of interest in his general ethnographic fieldwork. Thus Bateson demonstrated his thinking about children and how the relationship between children and adults goes to the heart of the dynamic of relationships in his book *Naven*, a text which has rarely been read by systemic psychotherapists in the UK or Europe (Bateson, 1958). Maria Esther and Britt have both long been interested in Bateson's ethnographic work related to children in New Guinea and in Bali. Maria Esther referred to Bateson's work with Balinese children in Chapter 3 in this book and the Naven ritual has been described in Chapter 4 by Britt. In both cases it was the relationship and the process of relating which was of interest to Bateson. In New Guinea the relationship between the mother's brother and the sister's son reaches a climax and is resolved, whereas in Bali a sequence of interaction in which a mother may begin a kind of flirtation with a child causing the child to become excited, the mother's attention would wander, she would brush off any physical attacks and show no anger at all (Bateson, 1972, pp. 112–113). Bateson suggested that instead of the climax familiar from the Naven ceremony, a sort of "continuing plateau of intensity" (Bateson, 1991, p. 113) would emerge and that this was in tune with other aspects of the Balinese ethos such as expressed in the Balinese disapproval of competition and rivalry and in Balinese musical composition. Deleuze and Guattari used this notion of "plateau" in their book *A Thousand Plateaus* referring to "continuous regions of intensity constituted in such a way that they do not allow interruption by any external termination, any more than they allow themselves to build toward a climax" (Deleuze and Guattari, 2013, p. 23 (2002, p. 26)).

We have two comments to make on these observations, one relating to the specificity of child care and the constitution of children, the other to the more general and theoretical significance of Bateson's observations of the way systemic psychotherapists may think about relationships, not as between total people/objects but as a unique way of relating to partial aspects of one's environment. The first comment relates to the anthropological context in which Bateson was working during the 1930s and 1940s. While Bateson was not interested in childhood as such, Margaret Mead, his wife at the time, together with other anthropologists had made childhood a focus for research in order to understand the influence of "culture" in the formation of personalities and personal outlooks. We are here referring to what has been termed the "Culture and Personality School" in American cultural anthropology, which was later discredited as a kind of cultural determinism, depicting whole cultures as personality types. While this critique was appropriate, those researchers also moved forward a much more nuanced understanding of child development and child care than had been the case previously. One of the main proponents of this school was Erik Erikson, who worked on Native American reservations in South Dakota, USA during the 1940s and 1950s (Erikson, 1950). Erikson pointed out that far from being delinquent and deluded, the Native Americans on the reservations were carrying on traditions and ways of thinking which had been integral to their earlier ways of life and their values before being colonized. His general point was that socialization channels individual persons towards becoming strong and successful individuals in particular situated contexts, which "fit with" but are not determined by the cultural context in which they take place. Erikson, a psychoanalyst, famously examined potty training and weaning amongst the Sioux Indians, and related the relaxed attitude to the giving away rather than retaining of property to the former, and the fierce self-mutilation Sioux hunters would undergo at the Sundance ceremony to the latter (Erikson, 1950, pp. 108ff). Erikson's model was in tune with Benedict's ideas of cultural standardization[9] and criticized for neglecting individual differences and for conveying a kind of fax model of culture. However, once it is accepted that goals for socialization are different in different cultures, we can no longer expect that the developmental routes to growing up successfully be limited to those expressed and propagated in capitalist Western societies as if these processes are "natural".

Erikson's work inspired subsequent work with children in anthropology. For example, working with the Kaluli of Papua New Guinea, a community in which being an orator is greatly valued, the Schieffelins were interested in how babies learn to speak (Schieffelin, 1976; Schieffelin, 1990). They found that not only are the theories mothers hold about baby speech vastly different from our own in that baby talk and interpretations to infants and toddlers should be avoided, but also that learning to talk is intimately connected with strategies for socialization involving mothers taking the role of both herself and the infant or toddler in both dyadic and triadic interactions. The point was, not perhaps surprisingly, that when children learn a language they also learn a language of learning of everything else, including cultural values. These processes are of course largely unconscious or to use the language of Bourdieu, doxic.[10] A final example of work developed from Erikson's insights is the work of Jean Briggs with a three-year-old Inuit girl (Briggs, 1998, summarized in Krause, 2014). In this work Briggs shows how the expression or cultural idiom of "*ungaalirit*" meaning "say *ungaa*", "to cry like a baby", "to feel deep attachment or longing", "to arouse the wish to be with another person" is used in everyday play and interaction to create cultural and emotional dilemmas, which the child has to solve in culturally acceptable ways, which in this case includes refraining from showing anger and acknowledging reflexive and mutual connections and dependence. *"Ungaalirit"* is a special kind of attachment. In each of these three examples socialization is shown to be specifically directed towards fostering qualities which are valued and useful in particular social contexts, entering into what Foucault refers to as "axes of subjectivation" (Deleuze, 2006 (2015)), an interiorization of the outside. This then is our first comment on Bateson's rather general observations on the differences between the Iatmul people and the Balinese: the specifics matter – child development and expectations of children are not the same.

Our second comment relates to the systemic implications of specific differences for relationships and for our understanding and working with them. If a child's development and the course of this development is attuned to overall cultural expectations and what it means to be a person, then this does not stop with the adults immediately surrounding the child, because these adults are themselves living in relationships which contain the specifics of their relationships to others (Cavagnis, 2009; Krause, 2002). Here the critique made by Fonagy and colleagues of Bowlby's model of attachment can provide a starting point (Fonagy et al., 1995). Bowlby's model assumed that when a child grows up she will use an internalized image of her carer and if this caregiver herself is capable of emotional attunement, this will help the child control conflict and distress (Bowlby, 1969). The revised model changes the emphasis from experience of behavior to experience of reflection. The child does not internalize an image of her carer's stance, rather the child internalizes an image of her carer's stance towards her, as a thinking, desiring, believing, feeling and reflecting creature. In other words, with the image of her carer comes an image of herself comprehended through her carer's stance to her. As Fonagy suggested it is not a question of an image at all, but a question of a process (Fonagy et al., 1995, p. 257). We consider this a useful critique, while at the same time too limiting. The analysis stays with dyads. However, what goes for the infant must also go for the carer. The carer too internalizes her own caregiver's image of her as a thinking, desiring, believing, feeling and reflecting creature and in any situation this comes to constitute an important part of her experience of herself. The same can be said about the caregiver's carer and his or her carer and so on. No individual can exist before the social relationships that connect him or her to other persons in this chain or in any other part of social life. Carers do not communicate or convey only their own views and they do not have experiences which are only private. So, if a mother is very much loved by her brother and this uncle also adores his nephew, meets with him often and gives him presents regularly, this will sooner or later become an aspect that influences the child's ideas of familial relationships. And if the mother lives in a society in which particular value is placed on the relationship between herself and her brother – they may for example have rights in each other's persons (bodily substances or property) – and by extension between her brother and her son, so that it would be a mother's expectation even before she has children that her brother will be closely involved (in everyday life or in rituals) in the upbringing of his nephew, this will have further and perhaps different effects on the child's orientation to family life, his dreams, his motivations, his intentions and his symptoms. This is the Iatmul situation in which the intensity of the relationship between a man and his nephew is demonstrated in the Naven ceremony. But there is no question that it only involves these two people because their relationship is an affirmation of other relationships such as that between a man and his sister, a man and his sister's husband, a woman and her son and a husband and wife, the father of the siblings, the mother of the siblings etc. As Bateson's ethnography shows the Naven ceremony also implicated a much wider group of people and ultimately all those who considered they have relationships with each other (Bateson, 1958). This, then, is our second and more theoretical comment: the relationships, which are signified by a child or any one person, contain a multiplicity of positions, a "reciprocal lace" (Cavagnis, 2009; Krause, 2002; Sluzki, 2009) and therefore a multiplicity of possibilities and partial connections (Strathern, 2004; Krause, Chapter 4 of this volume). As noted in our first comment, these possibilities and partial connections always contain specific empirical details. The process, on the other hand, is self-organizing and in this sense it is general. In it is implicated a combination of forces which are aimed at maintaining a stable state with a regulatory mechanism (leading to plateau) or limiting this stable state (leading to climax).

Subjectivation

In this multiplicity of positions, in this "reciprocal lace" how do we systemic psychotherapists want to conceptualize the child as a subject? How do we think about what happens with a child, with his/her existence from the beginning and during the process of living? Does he/she evolve? If we stay with the dichotomy of individual and society we cannot begin to conceptualize how a child grows and develops in particular situated contexts except by stipulating either that every child is an autonomous, individual agent, who can go anywhere and develop in any direction propelled by inherent individual inclinations, or that every child becomes a version of the same depending on the context the way Erikson, Mead and the researchers of the Culture and Personality School conceptualized child development, namely that every child will be a kind of a "fax model" of a personality best suited to a particularly situated cultural environment. Neither of these ideas is adequate for grasping the complexity of relationships developing in particular contexts. Instead life needs to be understood as an active process of differentiation not by individuals in isolation but by individuals in relationships and therefore in systems. The active process is precisely a differentiation (in relationships), which has the capacity for self-organization. Here we refer to Maturana and Varela's work on autopoiesis in which they emphasize the recursion involved in all life (Maturana, 1980; Maturana and Varela, 1994). The functioning of life is a dynamic self-production of living systems, in which the intensive individuation processes occur through self-organization. The differences in intensity set in motion flows of matter and energy, so that individuals have an openness and an ability to affect and be affected and to form heterogeneous assemblies with other individuals (animals, humans, biological organisms, artificial organisms etc.). In this vision of life, the human subject is conceptualized as part of a great ecology, a piece in a much more complex machine. The unit of analysis is an assemblage[11] itself. The subject is an emergence rather than a phenomenon in itself, it is an epiphenomenon, an emerging entity of multiplicities. In this view the subject must be conceptualized as intimately connected to their circumstances through what is frequently described as a process of subjectification, referring to two ideas: a social or political technique of governing individuals on the one hand and a possibility of self-articulation or self-care on the other. The two aspects are connected to the extent that any search for an internal essence is doomed to failure, since this will be based on forced distinctions. Following Foucault, we refer to this process as a process of subjectivation, "a critical ontology of ourselves as a historic-practical test of the limits we may go beyond, and thus as work carried out by ourselves upon ourselves as free beings" (Foucault, 1997, p. 316) rather than subjectification, and following Deleuze we understand this process of subjectivation as a permanent process of organization in chaos. Being does not imply agency with an exterior that is already given. Rather agency folds with partial aspects of that outside (the historico-practical) and in that fold and in its constant unfolding, it becomes individualizing and self-organizing by subjecting itself. In this way the process of subjectivation is a process of differentiation rather than of identification, because there is no other identity than difference and this is the essence of what exists. Echoing Bateson we may say that, that which exists, exists because it differs. Someone may say that "a life begins", but actually life began much earlier and will continue much later. We might say that "life is affirmed" or with the biologist Wilhelm Roux, that "a living being grows" by "absorbing" exteriority: "A plurality that has very diverse activities wants to 'preserve' itself, not as identical to itself, but as 'living – commanding – obeying – nourishing – growing'" (Pal Pelbart, 2008). We are singularity, a fold of the outside (Blanchot, 1987), but this is an outside that is not outside, in the sense of opposite to the inside. It is a withdrawal of forces on itself, the process through which the exterior constitutes the interior, which in turn will be constituted as a new mode of subjectivation. Deleuze explains: "The outside is not a fixed limit, but a moving matter animated by peristaltic movements, folds and foldings that together make up an inside: they are not something other than the outside, but precisely the inside of the outside" (Deleuze, 2006,

p. 80). In his lectures at Vincennes, Foucault proposed that Being results from the relations, oppositions and compromises between three dimensions, also in his last works referred to as the three ontologies: the ontology of knowledge, the ontology of power and the ontology of self. Knowledge-Being is determined by the visible and the articulable; Power-Being is determined within relations between forces and Self-Being is determined by the process of subjectivation, by "places crossed by the fold" (Deleuze, 2006, p. 94). Deleuze goes on to clarify,

> Given certain conditions they do not vary historically; but they do vary *with* history. What in fact they present is the way in which the problem appears in a particular historical formation: what can I know or see and articulate in such and such a condition for light and language? What can I do, what power can I claim and what resistances may I counter? What can I be, with what folds can I surround myself or how can I produce myself as a subject? On these three questions the "I" does not designate a universal but a set of particular positions occupied within a One speaks, One sees, One confronts, One lives.
>
> (Deleuze, 2006, p. 94)

The fold is a continuous process. It takes place in a historical context, which poses particular problems for particular selves. So for our clients who are refugees, for example, the problems faced are not only posed by the politics of the state, the inclusion and exclusion processes prominent at a particular time; they are also posed by lack of access to housing, health care and social relationships. Such a context was faced by Radia, a Tigrayan refugee, who was 26 years old when she was referred to the family service in which Britt worked. The reason this young woman had sought a referral from her General Practitioner was because she was not able to get pregnant. This was a rather unusual reason for referral; however, as the work developed Britt also learnt that Radia suffered from headaches, tightness in the body, nightmares, difficulty controlling her eating and that she often scratched herself on her arms and legs so she bled. During the work with Radia, a process of Radia struggling to produce herself as a subject also unfolded. Radia had experienced her father's murder in front of her when she was nine years old, after which her mother had left the extended family, driving away in a bus, while Radia was watching through the window. After a couple of years Radia fled Tigray, then in the grips of a very bloody three-way war between Ethiopia, Eritrea and Tigray, with her younger sister, who was disabled. The two girls fled over desert, dodging mines and eventually becoming separated amongst other refugees from this war. Radia found a place as a servant with a Saudi family who severely abused her. She described trying to drink bleach to end her life and feeling very desperate. The family moved to London and Radia absconded living in the streets for a couple of days, after which she was found in

Hyde Park[12] by a youth worker, who helped her register for benefits and find a place to live. This was several years before she was referred to the Family Service, at which point she was living with her Eritrean husband still in the same flat in social housing. During the next several years a process emerged in the therapy, which at several points taught Britt about the folding processes involved in Radia producing herself as a subject, the way the outside became the inside of her thoughts, feelings, intentions and aspirations and the places "crossed by the fold" in Radia's experiences of her life. The first time Britt began to grasp this was when Radia told her about the complex abusive situation in her extended family. After her mother had left Radia found herself living in her maternal family's house, but she was being treated as a servant, not given enough food and having to clean and carry firewood every day. Just before she ran away with her younger sister, she was accused of being a witch. The explanation of this from the point of view of Radia's maternal kin only emerged later and was this: Radia's maternal family and especially her maternal grandmother of some standing had planned for Radia's mother to marry into a particular family in Tigray with whom they already had ties. However Radia's mother had thwarted this wish and instead married a young radical lawyer, Radia's father. When he was killed by Ethiopian soldiers, Radia's mother and her four children continued to be shunned by her maternal family. Radia thought that the elopement of Radia's mother had been the justification for cutting her mother off from any inheritance and from denying her any sense of belonging and for the maltreatment of Radia and her siblings. This went as far as accusing Radia of witchcraft and, as Radia later explained to me, witches were considered anti-social forces excluded from the protection of moral communities and this accusation was one particularly leveled against infertile women. In telling this, it was clear that Radia felt ostracized, not just from the family home and the kinship group, but that she also felt prevented from being able to practice her own sense of relational personhood, self-care and self-making. In our work many years later this became one of the places crossed by the many folds in Radia's life. Radia and her Eritrean husband had four attempts at IVF, all of them unsuccessful. As a solution to Radia's predicament her husband suggested that he would take a second wife and this way Raida would have children to look after as his first wife and in this sense become a mother and a kinswoman. Radia felt outraged, doubly deprived and thwarted at this suggestion.[13] Eventually, Radia became a care assistant and when she recently telephoned Britt, she told her how she had looked after her sister who had been very ill and died in a London hospital. In sharing her story Radia taught Britt about the complex and often painful assemblage of ontological folds, which were the conditions for her emergent processes of subjectivation, in which the outside formed a co-extensive inside as illustrated by her burning wish to become pregnant. Radia's life did not begin with structure. It began, as does all life, with chaos in which the structure, the context and the environment are immanent, emerging and contingent, rather than being imposed from above, the inside or the outside.

Genograms or Cartography

Inspired by Deleuze and Foucault we have suggested that there are many interesting lines of enquiry to follow when we try to understand children and their relationships to the world around them. We suggested that, first, only one of these may relate to parentage, family, identity and attachment and, second, that parentage, family, identity and attachment as processes never stand alone but are implicated in complex processes of folding during which processes of subjectivation emerge. Despite the systemic psychotherapy tradition emphasizing "context" and the relationship between different systems, it is fair to say that when it comes to work in the clinic, systemic psychotherapists tend to begin with enquiring into the family and the parentage of the child. This is referred to as working with a genogram, a technique for which systemic psychotherapists have become famous and which has been exported to many social care departments in the UK at least. What is a genogram? Put succinctly, it is a format for drawing a family tree that records the information about family members and their relationships, taking into account at least three generations. Family therapists or systemic psychotherapists are not the only ones who use this kind of format. Social anthropologists, whose object of study for a long time remained focused on "kinship", "marriage" and "family", also draw up family trees and call these genealogies.[14] In both cases these two disciplines have agreed on constructing "the family" as an object of study, in this way institutionalizing the genogram or the genealogy as the most recurrent technique. However, both genogram and genealogy presuppose a theory, which explain the creation, the constitution and the composition of the object of study. In both cases this theory is that of the twentieth-century European family in which relationships (at least for official purposes) tended to be traced bilaterally and cognatically and which therefore appeared to consist of a naturally undifferentiated set of relatives and as a reflection of the way things really are in the natural (genetic) world. In social anthropology this model has received strong criticism for being middle-class and ethnocentric and responsible for erasing certain similarities in relationships between ethnographers and the people they traditionally studied (Bouquet, 1993; Krause, 1998; Strathern, 1992).[15] As far as family therapy is concerned, the first articles referring to genograms were published in the United States in 1976 and the interest in developing this tool and in training psychotherapists in how to use it to evaluate families increased from the end of the 1970s. In 1985, McGoldrick and Gerson published the first book on techniques in the use of genograms (McGoldrick and Gerson, 1989 (1985)). In this book they attempted to standardize the approach and it is this genogram model which is most generally used in contemporary systemic psychotherapy. In general the details taken into account for the preparation of the genogram are: family structure, both biological and legal; the registration of information (names, ages, occupations etc.), the type of relationships (merged, conflicting, separated, distant etc.), family roles; life events; family life cycle; family network context. In Argentina, Maria Rosa Glasserman further pioneered the development of work with the therapist's genogram as part of the family therapy training (Glasserman, 2007) and these practices are still important aspects of the curriculum for post-graduate students in systemic psychotherapy and family therapy in both the UK and Argentina.

It is easy to discern the influence of the dominant psychoanalytic paradigm in this account of the development of the genogram. For example the production of subjectivity tends to be considered to be a single mode of parenting, namely that found in the Western bourgeois nuclear family at the center of Freud's thinking about the Oedipus complex etc. Further, the genogram suggests that the family is a synonym for a system in this way limiting the context and the medium in which subjectivation occurs to the familiar and with it the possibility of accommodating other possible systems. The reading of the familiar becomes a structural reading and only refers to the biological family or variations on it. Finally, the genogram tends to depict and recognize relationships, which include hierarchical, linear and vertical descendants, whereas relationships between cognates and affine or other collateral kinship relationships tend to be left out.

In this way the genogram as a paradigm can be seen as having a constraining effect on the work of the therapist to such an extent that the therapist's ability and possibilities for thinking about relationships in a different way, of establishing other paths of enquiry, tend to be limited. The questions the therapist asks within this frame tend to refer back to the theory which generated the approach in the first place, and new, unique and surprising thoughts and practices will be noticed by the therapist only with difficulty. An alternative approach would be approaching relationships from the point of view of much more uncertain and unpredictable gestures in the therapy room, such as those we may describe as wandering, knitting, erring, travelling, straying or drifting. These are all verbs, which suggest the idea that nothing is given. Unlike following maps in a therapeutic space, they suggest the possibility of emergence of new and unique cartographic practices. In this idea, cartographies, unlike maps, are not given, they emerge at the same time as we cross the landscape. The difference between wandering through an unknown city and taking a tour is to allow something to happen, while it is happening. It is not about finding what already exists, nor what is sought, but of creating through the wander what is found. This entails getting rid of our maps and allowing ourselves to wander into new territories, to trace new paths and perhaps open new worlds of references. We say "getting rid" because the maps are in us, for example what appears as an error can be thought of as a clear indication that a map is operating, that we are not thinking, that we are imposing our own representations on the situation. It is necessary to be patient, not to crush an emergence with our theories and if the clients refuse our interpretations, to avoid attributing this to an effect of resistance or hostility.

In this we have been influenced by the ideas of Deligny who says: "Wandering is an infinitive that must remain as such, to preserve its extreme wealth, and it is only achieved to the extent that space remains vague, or must be 'unoccupied'" (Deligny, 2015b). Deligny was concerned with the dichotomization of subjectivities into normal and abnormal. He conducted a series of residential programs for children and adolescents with autism which he referred to as "attempts", searching for a way of being that would allow the children to exist without expecting any particular conception of humanity according to which no one subjectivity would be more dominant or normalized than another (Deligny, 2015a, p. 79). In 1967, he moved to the mountains of Cevennes, where he lived until his death in 1996. There he explored and developed his thoughts on cartography. The method is simple. He first drew a basic map of the landmarks of everyday life, such as the kitchen, the bathroom, the bedrooms, the water well etc. He then made a tracing on a sheet of transparent paper to track the movements made in space during the day. Thus, while the first map marks starting points, the second route consists of lines that map the movements of the so called "near presences", which indicate actions such as cooking or drawing water from the well. These lines were generally straight and practical. However there were also other lines that were curves, repetitive and going nowhere in particular. Deligny called these non-utilitarian lines, *ligne d'erre* (wandering lines) (Deligny, 2015a) a concept which later captured the attention of Deleuze and Guattari, particularly by the way in which a rhythm emerges from them (Deleuze, 1997 (1996)).

To think of the processes of subjectivation as cartographic is different from thinking of subjects who cross territories. Subjectivation occurs in the path, which is not present, but only emerges and is therefore linked to the idea of wandering and the idea of an event. The territory in cartography as a method is not given, but is that which is constructed as it is travelled. Neither is the subject given, there is no subject travelling a territory. "The territory is more than the organism and the environment, and the relationship between the two" (Deleuze and Guattari 2013, p. 504 (2002)). Just as the map is not the territory, the environment is not the territory. Chaos is the "environment of all environments" (Deleuze and Guattari 2013, p. 313 (2002)) and milieus, which should not be confused with territories, provide a certain safeguard against chaos. Deleuze and Guattari use the term "milieu" in at least three ways, which must be combined: 1) milieu refers to the environment or the ecosystem; 2) it refers to what is between two points, in the middle of a binary relationship; and 3) the term is used in science to refer to a substance that has the ability to transfer energy from one place or source to another and therefore denotes movement (Deleuze and Guattari, 2013, p. xvii (2002)).

Subjectivity, even though indistinguishable, is produced by three types of cartographic lines, the first two segmentary (stratification and chaos) and the third characterized by absolute deterritorialization (the chaos beneath and within territories): 1) the molar or the rigid line; 2) the molecular or flexible line recognized for its tendency to de-terriorialization; and 3) the line of flight that is not segmented (Deleuze and Guattrari, 2013, pp. 195–197 (2002)). The molar aspect indicates the main component of our lives and typically contributes to what we perceive as our identity, for example race, sex, gender, profession, nationality etc. The molecular aspect is more imperceptible, "travelling at speeds beyond the usual or ordinary thresholds of perception" (Deleuze and Guattari, 2013, p. 196 (2002)) and therefore can denote lines of deterritorialization that can produce variations in the molar organizations's network. The third type of lines, lines susceptible to variation and modification, become lines of flight. When we talk about territorialization/deterritorialization we refer to a relationship between organizing and disorganizing chaos or organization, not as opposed positions, but as processes present in the flow of vitality.[16] Guattari refers to a child singing in the night because "he fears the dark... and seeks to regain control of events that were de-territorialized too quickly" proliferating "on the side of the cosmos and the imaginary". Thus singing or rather returning to singing (as in the *ritornello* or Nietzsche's eternal return) allows an environment for the child to emerge from the chaos. It is not repetition, which produces difference through rhythm, because that would imply a structure already there, it is difference (or chaos) that is rhythmic, so that difference is substantive rather than a product. It is difference itself, which provides the child with something to hold on to. As in Bateson (1972, pp. 8–16), the difference is constitutive, which means that the rhythm arises from the difference between the singing and the return to singing, instead of the difference being produced in the interaction between the medium and the rhythm. Diversity is given, but difference is that by which something constantly differs. Everything that happens and everything that appears correlates with orders of differences: differences in level, temperature, pressure, tension potential, difference from intensity. In the cartographic work it is the opportunity of the appearance of a gesture that when amplified leads to deterriorialization, and it is possible to reterritorialize, to move from one to the other. Deleuze and Guattari explain the passage from one to the other as a movement from function to expression (Deleuze and Guattari, 2013 (2002, pp. 117–153)).

For us cartography adds a new dimension to our work with children and families in the clinic, because these ideas highlight not just paying attention to the present and what is happening in the therapy room between ourselves and our clients, but also because they alert us to the need to pay attention to the straight and wandering lines travelled in the space of the therapeutic context and how to pick up and not overlook unexpected gestures and stopping points which may highlight new processes or new aspects of processes and relationships. In good old-fashioned systemic terminology we may say that the ideas of cartography can help us be extra-specially attentive, stay with our curiosity and refrain from making assumptions based on what we already know.

Such wandering lines were shown to Britt in her work with Alfi and his parents. Alfi was an eight-year-old white English boy who lived with his mother Anita and his father Christopher. He was an only child and Christopher suffered from advanced Parkinson's disease. Both Anita and Christopher were writers, but Christopher could not work anymore and the family had regular help from an au pair and from hospital staff. Anita was central in managing daily life and she contacted the CAMHS service feeling that she could not manage Alfi. At first Alfi, Anita and Christopher all attended the outpatient clinic, even though this was often difficult for Christopher as his legs were badly affected by the disease and the optimum timing of his medication working did not always coincide with the best timing for Alfi in terms of missing school. Anita expressed her despair both at managing Alfi but also at managing the situation between the three of them. It turned out that Christopher did spend time with Alfi helping him with his school work, but that Alfi frequently was reluctant and the situation often ended with an argument in which Christopher found it very difficult to hold his position. For example, it happened that Alfi would kick Christopher's walking stick away from him, which made it impossible for Christopher to get out of his chair. It was very sad to hear Christopher talk about this in the session with mixed feelings, both of understanding for Alfi but also with grief of not being able to be the father he wanted to be. Anita, too, was in despair. However, in our session a slightly different picture emerged. When Britt and a trainee family therapist first met the family, Alfi, who did not want to talk at first, quickly turned to the whiteboard and began to write his answers, not once but several times, so that in the end there would be three versions of answers to trivial question such as: "Do you have a cat or a dog?" Alfi showed himself to be extremely good at writing and also at finding what might be behind a question. For example, he wrote "scary" when his mother told him off. Verbally he would also repeat an answer many times and do so while he moved rapidly around the room, at one point throwing himself at his father. In a subsequent session, which was conducted online due to the Covid-19 crisis, the air was full of repetitions from Alfi of words or lines which had been uttered by the adults, such as "everyday", "everyday", "everyday" and "lack of regularity", "lack of regularity" etc., "so true", "so true" and "bad goings on", "bad goings on", all the while Alfi was moving rapidly around the room behind his parents backwards and forwards, fetching his guitar and playing and coming back. Anita commented on this behavior being "a bit mad". We talked about this and Britt said that she felt a certain creativity in Alfi, which somehow embarrassed his mother, who talked about what other people might think and how odd she found Alfi's behavior. Eventually, we were able to have a conversation about what these repetitions and movements around the room might mean and Anita said that she felt that this was an outpouring of energy and vitality and that this in some way captured the opposite of Christopher's state, which was very still and sometimes came across as transfixed. These sequences reminded Britt of Guattari's statement quoted above and suggested how Alfi could find a milieu or an environment in chaos. Later the repetitions and the difference between them also became the focus for the future work with this family in which we began to understand these gestures better as a search for comfort and reassurance in returning to words, which because they were repeated, meant something new.

This difference between genogram and cartography was demonstrated to Maria Esther in her work with Ismael, a 40-year-old lawyer who was married to Virginia. Together they had one daughter aged four. Ismael sought help in order to work through a crisis: a year and a half before consultation he had had an affair with a 36-year-old workmate, Eva, who was married, with two children ages four and six. "I made a mistake", he said, "I'm a fool. I love my wife and daughter. They are everything to me! I just don't know what came over me... It was a new feeling, that a woman found me attractive..." Not long after that Eva told Ismael that she is pregnant... and he said: "That was the end of the world. I risked losing what I valued most, my family. I was being punished. I tried to persuade Eva to have an abortion but she wouldn't hear of it. She wanted that baby and said she would raise it as her own. She had told her husband and they had agreed I was to be banished from their lives forever".

Ismael told his wife Virginia six months after the boy's birth. The news was deeply unsettling to her. She said that she could not live with the thought that the man she had married should just give up a child of his. She said, "I don't know you, You are not the man I married...". Ismael insisted that he felt no bond to the child. He said, "It's just as if I had been a sperm donor". The therapy did not go on for long after that. The client and Maria Esther had gone over and over assumptions and beliefs: that fatherhood is a biological event, a sociocultural construction. They explored the nature of desire and although, as a lawyer, Ismael knew DNA testing would give him grounds to claim the baby as his own, he chose not to take legal action in the certainty that the truth would be of no use to anyone concerned. As for herself, Maria Esther, the therapist, was left in uncertainty, fully aware of the complexity of the matter at all sorts of levels: the child's right to know his/her origin; fatherhood as a social bond arising from desire; theories on the psychological effects of concealment on the one hand, and the marks left in the process of subjectivation by the father's rejection on the other. Many of these questions Maria Esther shared with Ismael during his treatment.

As a young university student in Argentina, Maria Esther witnessed the pain and suffering caused by the state of terror, when mothers came together as Mothers of Plaza de Mayo seeking to know the fate of their disappeared children, and later, when those grieving women, as grandmothers, Abuelas of Plaza de Mayo, sought to restore the identities of the children born to the disappeared in captivity, torn away from their mothers at birth and appropriated by members of the armed forces and others (see also Chapter 4 in this book). Over time, forensic anthropology and genome analysis have provided material evidence of the crimes of the dictatorship: many of the remains of the disappeared have been identified. DNA testing has also enabled a number of those children to gain access to their biological origin and thus meet the families and their kin. Many of them, driven by a deeply felt, unfathomable unconscious sense of the unspoken, have as adults chosen to know the truth, which, in some cases, such as Estela Carlotto's[17] grandson, has meant a new valuation of their bond with their foster family, who had no knowledge of their origins. The disclosure of the biological identities of these children, however, has not always led to a happy ending for them. Many of Maria Esther's contemporaries have been confronted by those events in their practice, the older generation, through lived experience, the younger ones, through the effect of the transgenerational memory of sorrow and pain. Regardless of ideology, those events live on in our memory, folded into our cultural subjectivity.

So, let us imagine the child born to Ismael and Eve, brought up by Eve and Edward as their own, as an eight-year-old today, in therapy, diagnosed as suffering from learning difficulties. One therapist might focus on the genogram of his acknowledged parents, while another might attempt to delve into and bring together the two stories, the official one and the other, the secret, untold story of his biological origin. Which would be the geno-gram of choice? How to avoid the limitations of our ontological givens? Mapping is the only way. Cartography will enable us to follow the signs along the trajectory that emerges in the clinic, blindfolded though alert to the unexpected revelation of the event that triggered the symptom. What unfolds is a unique path unlike any other child's. Cartography, when suc-cessful, is the means to an end that may enable the child's parents to remove the obstacles and release a new force.

Concluding Remarks

In this chapter we have suggested that systemic psychotherapeutic work with children offers an opportunity to take forward our work with differ-ence, that is taking forward the placing of difference at the heart of how we perceive ourselves and our clients in our work. This does not only involve working with differences in terms of race, gender, class, culture, ethnicity, age etc., but working with difference with all clients at all times. We have tried to point to a perspective critical of traditional psychology, family therapy and child psychotherapy by considering the political, ethical and aesthetic aspects of work with children. We were able to do so because of the unique revolutionary and inventive aspects of childhood and the opportunities these offer to psychotherapists looking to critique the status quo in both theory and practice. In putting together our thoughts and practice we have been inspired by the thinking of Bateson, Deleuze and Guattari, Foucault, Strathern, and others, and we offered four general points. First, we showed how attachment theory tends to reproduce normative expectations derived from Western notions of the family and family relationships and tends to close down the possibility that children communicate other wider relationships and concerns including those derived from wider political and ecological contexts. Second, we argued that "reality" is an effect, that is to say we see "reality" as an emergence of relationships and practices and we used cross-cultural examples of attachment to develop this point. Our analysis required a theory of multiplicity in relationships, of partial connections, of a reciprocal lace and an appreciation of "what lies behind". In this sense our argument is a plea for the affirmation of uniqueness against assumptions about what is universal. The process itself, however, is self-organizing and therefore general, leading to a climax as in Bateson's work on the Naven ceremony or to a plateau as in Balinese childcare, as was picked up by Deleuze and Guattari. Third, we considered the child as a subject and subjectivation as an active process of differentiating the subject. We drew on Foucault's writing on the process of folding in subjectification and we considered the unit of analysis to be an "assemblage", that is to say an emerging collective containing a number of different elements, material and non-material, rather than individuals or individual events. In this we are placed firmly in an ontology of difference and becoming, with an emphasis on process rather than "essences". Finally, we turned our attention to what these observations mean for how we work with children as systemic psychotherapists. We do not dispute that genograms have been and still can be useful in working psychotherapeutically in systemic psychotherapy. However, we also suggest that genograms in particular and the way these are used in psychotherapeutic sessions suffer from many of the shortcomings we have critiqued in this chapter. We therefore propose a complementary approach in the notion of cartography, inspired by the work of Deligny. We suggested that by tracing movement, repetition and differences in the therapy sessions we may achieve several new ways of viewing our work. First, this pays attention to micro-processes in the therapeutic session and is in line with the best traditions of systemic psychotherapeutic practice. Second, in considering the gestures and movements in the therapy session as "wandering lines" following Deligny, we are pointing to lines defying prescription and ideology unveiling unexpected gestures and stopping points, which might highlight new processes. In this we have been inspired by the work of Deleuze and Guattari and the notions of molar, molecular lines as well as the idea of "lines of flight" directing our attention to the ever present possibility of something new emerging for our clients and ourselves in our work. Finally, we have suggested that the concept of "context" itself needs to be examined in relation to processes of subjectivation and the folding which this process implies. We have suggested that context must be thought of not as something given, but as those specific and partial aspects with which it relates.

Notes

1 The two authors have made use of editions in respectively English and Spanish. When both editions of a work are referred to, the first reference is to the English edition and the second to the Spanish edition.
2 Radcliffe-Brown was Bateson's supervisor during his work with the Iatmul in New Guinea.
3 In reference to dynamic systems, a fork occurs when a variation in the values of the parameters of a system causes an abrupt "qualitative" or topological change in its behavior. Balance changes in any of the invariants cross critical thresholds. See also Maturana (1980) and Maturana and Varela (1994).
4 The notion of unity only appears when in a multiplicity there is a seizure of power by the signifier, or a corresponding process of subjectivization. The unit always acts within an empty dimension supplementary to that of the system considered (over-coding). But precisely a rhizome or multiplicity is not allowed to codify.
5 Here Deleuze is referring to a well-known case, that of Little Hans written about by Freud.
6 "Machines refer to institutions, social arrangements and psychological and biological systems. The function of machines can be understood as either connective, disjunctive or conjunctive and working together these operations allows for other processes such as production, recording and enjoying" (Deleuze and Guattari, 2004, pp. 2–27 (1980, pp. 11–18)). See also Krause referring to the work of Marilyn Strathern in Chapter 4 of this volume.
7 Deleuze and Guattari refer to this as "body without organs" (1980, pp. 18–24, 2013, pp. 180–198).
8 With transcendence explanations privilege one substance at the expense of another, whereas with immanence substances are produced while remaining in themselves (see May, 2005).
9 Ruth Benedict and her idea of standardization influenced Bateson, Mead, Erikson and others of the Culture and Personality School (Benedict, 1934).
10 "*Doxa*" refers to "thoughts" or predispositions and "habitus" to the structuring structure which influences the formation of such predispositions (Bourdieu, 1990).
11 "Assemblage" refers to non-personal multiplicities in which "the mode of individuation of 'a life' does not differ in nature from that of 'a climate', 'a wind', 'a fog' or 'an hour of the day'" (Smith, 1997, p. xxxiv). "We are not in the world, we become with the world, we become by contemplating it" (Deleuze and Guattari, 1991, p. 169).
12 One of central London's large and popular parks.
13 Polygamy is traditionally a way of addressing the problem of childlessness in certain cultures.
14 Family therapy uses symbols also employed in genetics, whereas social anthropology traditionally uses triangles instead of squares for men and different connecting symbols.

15 For example the traditional assumption that English Middle classes are "kinship-less", which is echoed in the tacitly expressed view that "culture" and "ethnicity" are something ascribed to minority populations only.
16 Deleuze and Guattari refer to vitality as "a force that is, but does not act" (Deleuze , 1994, p. 213). There are many other concepts involved in their thinking about the processes outlined above and we refer the reader to their publications, in particular Gilles Deleuze, *Difference and Repetition* and Gilles Deleuze and Felix Guattari, *A Thousand Plateaus*. Here we are limit ourselves to refer to concepts, which we find are necessary to show how the cartography may add to our therapeutic thinking and our uses of genograms.
17 Estela Barnes de Carlotto is an Argentinean human rights activist and President of the Abuelas de Plaza de Mayo association.

References

Bateson, G. (1958). *Naven: The Culture of the Iatmul People of New Guinea as Revealed Through a Study of the "Naven" Ceremonial*. London: Wildwood House.

Bateson, G. (1972). *Steps to An Ecology of Mind. Collected Essay in Anthropology, Psychiatry, Evolution, and Epistemology*. London: Jason Aronson.

Bateson, G. (1991). *A Sacred Unity. Further Steps to An Ecology of Mind*. R.E. Donaldson (ed.). London: Harper Collins.

Benedict, R. (1934). *Patterns of Culture*. New York: Houghton Miflin Company.

Bergson, H. (1960). *Time and Free-Will: An Essay on the Immediate Data of Consciousness*. New York: Harper & Row.

Bertalanffy, L. (1969). *General Systems Theory: Foundations, Developments and Applications*. New York: George Braxiller.

Bertalanffy, L. (1976). *Teoria general de los sistemas*. Mexico City: Fondo de Cultura Económoca.

Blanchot, M. (1987). Michel Foucault as I imagine him. In *Foucault/Blanchot*. New York. Zone Books.

Bouquet, M. (1993). *Reclaiming English Kinship: Portuguese Refractions of British Kinship Theory*. Manchester: Manchester University Press.

Bourdieu, P. (1990). *The Logic of Practice*. Cambridge: Polity Press.

Bourdieu, P. (1998). The family spirit. In *Practical Reason: On the Theory of Action*. Cambridge: Polity Press.

Bowlby J. (1969). *Attachment and Loss*, Vol 1. New York: Basic Books.

Briggs, J.L. (1998). *Inuit Morality Play: The Emotional Education of a Three-Year Old*. New Haven, CT: Yale University Press.

Byng-Hall, J. (1995). *Rewriting Family Scripts: Improvisation and Systemic Change*. New York, CT: The Guilford Press.

Cavagnis, M.E. (2009). Los cuentos que nos contamos los terapeutas de niños. *Revista sistemas familiares y otros sistemas humanos*, 1, 24–36.

Cavagnis, M.E. (2014). Nuevos padres, nuevos hijos, nuevas formas de ser hacer familia. *Redes y Paradigmas*, 8, 137.

Dallos, R. and Draper, R. (2005). *An Introduction to Family Therapy: Systemic Theory and Practice*. Maidenhead: Open University Press.

Deleuze, G. (1994). *Difference and Repetition*. London: Bloomsbury.

Deleuze, G. (1996). Lo que dicen los niños. In *Crítica y clínica*. Barcelona: Anagrama.

Deleuze, G. (1997). What children say. In *Essays, Critical and Clinical*. Minneapolis, MN: University of Minnesota Press.

Deleuze, G. (2006). *Foucault*. London: Bloomsbury.

Deleuze, G. (2014). *El Bergsonismo*. Buenos Aires: Cactus.

Deleuze, G. (2015). *La subjetivación: curso sobre Foucault*. Buenos Aires: Cactus.

Deleuze, G. and Guattari, F. (1980). *El antiedipo: capitalismo y esquizofenia*. Buenos Aires: Paidos.

Deleuze, G. and Guattari, F. (1991). *What is Philosophy?* New York: Columbia University Press.

Deleuze, G. and Guattari, F. (2002). *Mil mesetas, capitalismo y esquizofrenia*, 5th edn. Valencia: Pre-Textos.

Deleuze, G. and Guattari, F. (2004). *Anti-Oedipus: Capitalism and Schizophrenia*. London: The Athlone Press.

Deleuze, G. and Guattari, F. (2008). La geologia de lo moral. In *Mil mesetas: capitalismo y esquizofrenia*. Valencia: Pre-Textos.

Deleuze, G. and Guattari, F. (2013). *A Thousand Plateaus*. London: Bloomsbury.

Deligny, F.B. (2015a). *Lo arácnido y otros textos*. Buenos Aires: Cactus.

Deligny, F.B. (2015b). *Vagabundos eficaces*. Barcelona: Universitat Oberta de Catalunya.

Elkaïm, M. (1990). *If You Love Me, Don't Love Me: Constructions of Reality and Change in Family Therapy*. New York: Basic Books.

Erikson, E. (1950). *Childhood and Society*. New York: W.W. Norton & Company.

Fonagy, P., Gergely, G., Jurist, E.L. and Tarjet, M. (2004). *Affect Regulation, Mentalization and the Development of the Self*. London: Karnac Books.

Foucault, M. (1997). *Ethics*, Vol. 1. *Essential Works of Foucault 1954–1984*. P. Rabinow (ed.). New York: The New Press.

Fraiberg, S. (1975). Ghosts in the nursery: A psychoanalytic approach to the problem of the impaired infant-mother relationship. *Journal of the American Academy of Child Psychiatry*, 14(3): 387–421.

Freud, S. (1918). The wolf man: From the history of infantile neurosis. In *The Standard Edition*, Vol. 17. pp. 1–124.

Freud, S. (1976). El hombre de los lobos: De la historia de una neurosis infantil. In *Obras completes*, Vol. 17. Buenos Aires: Amorrortu.

Glasserman, M.R. (2007). *Familias gravemente perturbadas*. Buenos Aires: Lugares.

Guattari, F. (2013). *Lineas de fuga*. Buenos Aires: Cactus.

Guattari, F. (2015). *Lines of Flight: For Another World of Possibilities*. London: Bloomsbury.

Haley, J. and Hoffman, L. (1967). *Terapia para resolver problemas*, 3rd edn. New York: Basic Books.

Haley, J. and Hoffman, L. (1968). *Techniques of Family Therapy*. New York: Basic Books.

Klein, M. (1932). *The Psychoanalysis of Children*. London: The Hogarth Press.

Klein, M. (1950). *El psicoanalisis de niños*, 1st edn. Buenos Aires: Paidos.

Koffman, O. (2015). Una persona más saludable y más eperanzada: ilegimidad, trastorno mental y er majhor pronóstico de las madres adolescentes. *Journal of Medical Humanities*, 36, 113–126.

Krause, I.-B. (1998). *Therapy across Culture*. London: Sage Publications.

Krause, I.-B. (2002). *Culture and System in Family Therapy*. London: Karnac Books.

Krause, I.-B. (2012). *Culture and Reflexivity in Systemic Psychotherapy. Mutual Perspectives*. London: Karnac Books.

Krause, I.-B. (2014). The complexity of cultural competence. In F. Lowe (ed.), *Thinking Space: Promoting Thinking about Race, Culture, and Diversity in Psychotherapy and Beyond*. London: Karnac Books.

LeVine, R.A. (2014). Teoría del apego como ideología cultural. In *Diferentes caras del apego: variaciones culturales sobre una necesidad humana universal*. Cambridge: Cambridge University Press.

LeVine, R.A., Dixon, S., LeVine, S., Richman, A., Leiderman, P.H., Keefer, C. and Brazelton, T.B. (1996). *Child Care and Culture: Lessons from Africa*. Cambridge: Cambridge University Press.

Madanes, C. (1981). *Strategic Family Therapy*. San Francisco, CA: Jossey-Bass.

Madanes, C. (1984). *Terapia familiar estratégica*. Buenos Aires: Amorrortu.

Maturana, H. and Varela, F. (1994). *De máquinas y seres vivos*, 1st edn. Santiago: Universitaria S.A.

Maturana, U. (1980). *Autopoiesis and Cognition: The Realisation of Living*. Boston: D. Reidel.

May, T. (2005). *Gilles Deleuze: An Introduction*. Cambridge: Cambridge University Press.

McGoldrick, M. and Gerson, R. (1985). *Genogramas en la evaluación familiar*. Barcelona: GEDISA.

McGoldrick, M. and Gerson, R. (1989). Genograms and family life cycle. In B. Carter and M. McGoldrick (eds), *The Changing Family Life Cycle*. Boston, MA: Allyn and Bacon.

Minuchin, S. (1974). *Families and Family Therapy*. London: Tavistock Publications.

Minuchin, S. (2003). *Familias y terapia familiar*, 8th edn. Barcelona: Gedisa.

Morin, E. (1981). *El método I: La naturaleza de la naturaleza*. Madrid: Catedra.

Morin, E. (1990). *Introducción al pensamiento complejo*. Barcelona: Gedisa.

Oakley, A. (1971). *Sujeto Mujeres*. Oxford: Martin Robertson.

Pakman, M. (1994). Introducción. In *Introduccion al pensamiento complejo*. Barcelona: Gedisa.

Pal Pelbart, P. (2008). Cartografias del afuera. *Collège international de Philosophie | Rue Descartes*, 1(59), 20–30.

Prigogine, B. (1983). *¿Tan sólo una ilusión?* Barcelona: Tusquets.

Quinn, N. and Mageo, J.M. (2013). *Attachment Reconsidered: Cultural Perspectives on a Western Theory*. New York: Palgrave Macmillan.

Rodriguez Muñoz, M. (2020). Los padres de los rugbiers, los otros culpables. *Perfil*, 26 February, p. 8.

Schieffelin, B. (1990). *The Give and Take of Everyday Life: Language Socialisation of Kaluli Children*. Cambridge: Cambridge University Press.

Schieffelin, E.L. (1976). *The Sorrow of the Lonely and the Burning of the Dancers*. New York: St Martin's Press.

Sluzki, C. (2009). Bebes dificiles, progenitores dificieles: hacia un modelo basico en la calibración reciproca. *Redes*, 22, 11–27.

Smith, D.W. (1997). Introduction. "A life of pure immanence": Deleuze's "Critique et Clinique" Project. In G. Deleuze. *Essays Critical and Clinical*. Minneapolis, MN: University of Minnesota Press.

Strathern, M. (1992). *After Nature: English Kinship in the Late Twentieth Century*. Cambridge: Cambridge University Press.

Strathern, M. (2004). *Partial Connections*, updated edn. Oxford: Altamira Press.

Thom, R. (1977). *Stabilité structurelle et morphogénèse*. Paris: Interédition.

Vertere, A. and Dowling, E. (2016). *Narrative Therapy with Children and their Families*. London: Routledge.

Watzlawick, P. and Beavis, J.D. (1991). *Teoria de la comunicación humana*. Barcelona: Herder.

Watzlawick, P. and Beavis, J.D. (1997). *Pragmatics of Human Communication*. New York: W.W. Norton & Company.

Wilson, J. (1998). *Child-Focused Practice: A Collaborative Systemic Approach*. London: Karnac Books.

Chapter 7

Clinical Practice as Ecological Aesthetics

Pietro Barbetta, Maria Esther Cavagnis, Inga-Britt Krause and Umberta Telfener

Our group, the four of us, is multilingual, since we come from different countries, we speak different languages, we have different mother-tongues even when we speak the same language. Our usual work as clinicians is multilingual too: in therapy we try to act in the knowledge of the coexistence of multiple languages. The language of the psyche – among the many – emerges in the space between visible and invisible, between said, seen and acted. Beyond the tradition of *clinical work*, it is necessary to be curious about *how it works*. What is the machination that makes the clinics clinical? How "the clinic" connects its organs? Do the clinical organs have a clinical organism, under which they should be ordered? Or, maybe the clinic, in psychotherapy, has a rhizomatic connection, which frequently goes out from the clinical territory, investing the social, the cultural and the natural, as three sides of a same coin? What part does the unforeseen, the unpredictable event play? To answer these questions, and others that can rise from complexity, we need to revise our way of looking at clinics, taking distance from the capitalistic machine and the subsequent colonial positionings. We need to take into account that the clinics of the psyche are composed of human and non-human factors, and that a different relationship between persons and material objects – artifact or natural – produces the reality we are confronted with in our work (Barad, 2003).

Analysis of a Clinical Example

Let us analyze the following aspects of a so-called "clinical case", step by step, to find what is traditionally considered improper for the clinician, even though it occurs inside the clinics. Anna[1] is a 40-year-old woman who has many problems. She lives by herself with a three-year-old daughter and is afraid that her daughter could be taken away by social services as her work as a house cleaner has diminished and sometimes she doesn't have enough food for both of them. What people around her say has influence and her neighbors don't seem to like her, she is quarrelsome and her daughter often cries. The laws and the prejudices of the systems she is involved in seem

DOI: 10.4324/9780429437410-7

"against" her. Is she right in her judgment or a little paranoid? In the session she tells the therapist that she is coming to a public mental health clinic, after the neighbors reported her to the court. The therapist needed to deal not only with her psychic aspects but also with the housing issues, with the money she earns, how she spends it, what happens in the dark moments, and what happens when Anna feels ok.

We need to consider the economical and juridical aspects: the request from the court for the public institution to evaluate her, the issues brought forth by the social services and by other professionals who are now in contact with her. How is her housing situation, is she on welfare, where and with whom does her daughter stay; many are the questions we need to ask, considering many different aspects that interact very tightly with the emotional sphere. The events Anna talks about are not causes of predictable effects, they are rather undeterminable parts of the world in its becoming. She is part – and us as well – of the continuous reconfiguration of her world.

First issue: *clinical impoverishment*. Immediately the "pure clinician" thinks: this is a job for social workers, splitting Anna's social problems off from the clinical discourse (Foucault, 2008), while we think the story told until now has a vital influence on Anna's life.

Has Anna's impoverishment something to do with the clinic? Is it part of her psyche? Is impoverishment a symptom? Although poverty is not considered by the DSM, impoverishment seems to work like depression or other similar disorders described by any theoretical clinical handbook; day by day less work to be done, less salary, less food, as in depression, day by day less energy, less joy and more sadness. Nonetheless poverty is usually considered in the social domain and depression in the psychic one, an epistemological/ontological mistake since these two spheres are not separated.

Moreover, depressed people can usually afford themselves to pay the therapist, poor people cannot, and psychotherapy is supposed to be *honored*; as an Italian Marxist psychoanalyst – Elvio Facchinelli (1983) – ironically wrote: the salary of the psychotherapist is called "honorarium".

Who around Anna has some influence? Her neighbors do not seem to like Anna, she is quarrelsome and her daughter often cries. The prejudices of the systems in which she is involved seem "against" her.

Second issue: *clinical suspect*. Is Anna right in her judgment or a bit paranoid? One of the secondary symptoms of poor people, beyond poverty, is marginalization, which brings the reaction of protest from the part of whom is marginalized, and the counter reaction of the others: the accusation of being quarrelsome or even paranoid comes easily, and, with the accusation, the consequences. Such a situation can evolve in what Pietro in Chapter 2 calls "radial delirium": everybody who belongs to the community – neighborhood, palace, village – talks about it, gossip, moral disdain, aggression, even violence.

The economical, communitarian and juridical aspects involved within the clinic have to be assembled into the clinical practice and sometimes just one professional is not enough, a team should work together, despite the cost. The request from the court for the public institution to assess Anna's conditions; the issue brought forth by social services and by the other professionals who are now in contact with her; the social disapproval she gets from the community. How is her housing situation, is she on welfare, where does her daughter stay and with whom when she is at work, which places does she take her daughter to play, who else does the daughter interact with, are all relevant issues in the therapy room.

Third issue: *who is the customer, which is the mandate and from whom does it come*? Anna is seen at the mental health public clinic, sent by the court to make a diagnosis, the customer is the court and Anna is forced to come in order to state her positioning and try to demonstrate her good faith with her daughter. The professional in the public institute needs to elicit the need from Anna and to create her quest for the consultation. If she doesn't do so, the professional risks making the request very ambiguous and confusing the customer, therefore annulling the mandate. Is there an explicit quest on Anna's part? Does she want to be here with the professional of the public service or is she just afraid the judges could take her daughter away?

Fourth issue: *which positioning must the professional take*. Professionals have to take many positionings and are given many from their clients. In this case there are – as we said – material matters and psychic ones imbricated and there is the risk for Anna to be undermined and made weaker by the consultation. We also know that the therapeutic intervention is not a political one even if the professional cannot be neutral and needs to be aware of the political and social implications of what is happening.

Fifth issue: *how not to become "doctor homeostat", how not to collude and stop the inevitable evolution of any system, blocking its flow*. We will not deal with this issue here since it is clearly stated in Chapter 5, in which Umberta specifies that since we are inevitably ignorant and blind to some (not all) aspects of others we could not see that we don't see and therefore intervene within the dominant presuppositions with which the system is already functioning and maintain the homeostasis.

Sixth issue: *from whom is the problem-determined system formed and how do the different ideas on the problem maintain the status quo or create an evolutive process?* There are many professional figures sharing the same narration: social workers, psychologists, teachers, general doctors, neighbors, a judge, the social services, now also the mental health clinic and the professional's supervisor. It is impossible that they share all the same point of view and it is not even necessary; the clinician needs to know that these differences exist and needs to monitor if the process that is going on is evolutive or getting stuck, if there is a dominant hypothesis that reifies the status quo or there is space for differences.

All these questions, and possible others, are important, different aspects that tightly interact with the emotional sphere. Because feelings are not separable and dis-connectable from the materiality of things, artifacts, institutions, jobs, environments we live by, the subject is not just the interiority of "the Self" – whatever this word can mean – it is rather a network of all the issues mentioned above. As a human, Anna is part of the world in its becoming, she is part – and the therapist and the supervisor as well – of the continuous reconfiguration of their world.

The Evidence of the Material World: Ethic and Aesthetic

Why plan to bring back the material world into psychotherapy. Is not psychotherapy a therapy of the soul by definition? The recent upheaval of the world, including the viruses we recently faced – the Covid-19 is the last of a series – is bringing millions of people to their death; the planet warming, evidently due to human action; the new aggressive political panorama inside countries all over the world; the decreasing of fertility in post-capitalist and post-communist countries; and other important phenomena of the Anthropocene – all these elements mark the definitive sunset of linguistic-turn philosophical approaches. The materiality of the world out there has come back. What does the Antropocene mean for therapy?

Therapy needs a different approach, in which ethic and aesthetic matter more and more. Let us try to clarify once again, in this book, what we mean with "ethic" and "aesthetic".

Ethic is different from both moral and juridical, which does not mean being against moral or juridical. It means that moral has to do with the habits of social and communitarian life, it derives from the Latin word *mos*, meaning *habitude, uses, the usual way people live*, which varies from time to time and between different communities. A moral attitude brings about right and wrong judgment and the risk of thinking there are right or wrong actions to perform. The moral stance risks falling into fundamentalism, that claims that there are opposite ways of living. Or believing that "*our*" habits are the only affordable way to live, or considering any kind of habit a simple variable of "cultural normality", justifying human rights violations – such as infibulation, voodoo practices, woman oppression and other forms of body violation – as cultural variables.

If one confuses moralilty and ethics, one puts communitarian customs and habits as transcendental universal principles, such as for example: how women must dress, how men should behave, how children have to be raised, etc. As happens in totalitarian states, ethics and morality collapse into juridical laws, for example laws which forbid women to travel alone, to attend university courses, to drive, to divorce etc.

Ethics requires a suspension of the moral and the juridical; ethics suspends the abstraction made by the moral and juridical, it comes back to the immanence of a few principles such as "do not harm anyone", "respect the dignity of the other", "live honestly", which are included in the Heinz von Foerster (1984) imperative quoted above. Von Foerster used to say that ethics cannot be spoken because it immediately becomes a moralistic stance. Ethics emerges instead from the actions and the positioning the person chooses to enact, since ethics has two "sisters" that make her evident, though outspoken, and that express where it stands: the epistemological stance one chooses and therefore the attitude and the language one speaks, the respect shown in the relationship with the other. Ethics deals with the aesthetical shape of life, it deals with events as extraordinary and unforeseen, what in this book and in reference to complexity we call singularity. Ethics – as mercy, in the verses of Shakespeare – "seasons justice".

The word "aesthetic" comes from the Greek word *aisthesis*, that has multiple meanings, including: sensation, perception, feeling, from intellect as well as from senses, even scent; also discernment, as the one used to discern about ethics. For the antiques, ethic requires aesthetic as criterion, a particular kind of judgment. The materiality of the object makes the difference: is the object clear or obscure? Hard or soft? Intimate or estimable? Is it still or living? Is the object a body, or a part of it, an organ? The material world has a big part in the complex interconnection between ethic and aesthetic and all of this is not reducible to language. Bodies matter not just in the performative speech, they occupy a space, they move from here to there, they feel pain and grief etc. Therapy deals with materiality, which signifies units of movement that do not imply the primacy of language. At the same time, we do not think that language is representational: words are not necessarily mirroring pre-existing phenomena, objects are not pre-existing and independent from the emergence that occurs as a consensual, reciprocal, recursive coordination of coordination of consensual actions (Maturana and Varela, 1980).

What Meaning Do We Give to Symptoms

Symptoms express what is happening, they do not have a single function. Symptoms show something; as in Heraclitus, symptoms neither reveal nor conceal, they give signs.

As in Anna's case there is no hegemony of a central signifier: poverty, marginality, communitarian rejection, psychiatric services, juridical intervention, all these issues are assembled and concur in transforming the life of a woman who is losing her job into a person who faces hell. During the therapeutic process symptoms receive temporarily an unstable and hypothetical sense. Complexity, in clinical practice, consists in different kinds of hypothetical assemblages, in bricolaging parts in different ways. As in Anna's story, the time of the fabula can follow the time of the narrative, as in the mainstream: less job – poverty – less food for the child – child guidance intervention – quarrel – communitarian rejection – psychiatric hospitalization. What other assemblage of issues can one hypothesize for changing the meaning of this narrative? If we start at the end and go into the reverse direction, what happens? Psychiatric hospitalization – communitarian rejection – quarrel – child guidance intervention – less food for child – poverty – less job. Assembling the issues in reverse, one faces the strange loop of the escalation, the fulfilling prophecy of psychiatry labeling, which makes the links between the items stronger. Are there other chances? Can therapy increase the number of choices re-assembling the mentioned issues in different ways and redefining the signifiers? For example: therapy can shift the signifier "quarrel" into "protest", which can highlight the totalitarian part of our democracies. If one starts from protest, the totalitarian actions of being rejected by the community, forbidden to love and raise her child, being hospitalized as paranoid, becomes evident. This could be defined as a redefinition of "quarrel". The therapist, now, can take position besides Anna and what in systemic therapy has been called "joining" acquires a new and different sense – not just feeling "empathy", it is sharing with her a different voice, no more quarrels – the therapist has to protest, transforming therapy into a micro political issue.

This does not mean at all that the therapist has to become a solicitor or a syndicalist for Anna. Complexity does not require antagonism nor taking sides. Solicitors and labor union people substitute the subject, they put themselves in the place of the subject, a phenomenon of anthropophagy; they would repeat the violation of Anna's dignity in other ways. Solicitors tend to restore the political agenda of escalation; in such a case the protest would become counter-power – "contro potere", another way of bribery, a power alternative to power – and new corruption would take place. Can a minute, small little question – like a primrose being a joy forever – change Anna's life script? For example: "How it happens that, when you manifest your discontent, people tend to think that you are quarreling?" or "Is there anyone between your neighbors, medical doctors, social workers of judges who is listening to your quarrel?" with the confidence that even within the most ferocious dictatorship, there is always more than one discontent. It is what William Blake (1997) and Bateson (1972) call the "minute particular", a multidimensional architecture of concepts, not organized from the outside, but rather by the potential reach and the richness of intuit.

Nonetheless, we recommend the reader not to take this example too seriously, we are just proposing hypotheses. We could equally well start from another issue, for example from changing the lemma "loss of food" into "starving", and find other paths, such as the urgency to ask for charity. When we talk about "redefinition", we are not just playing with words, or imposing our words on the so-called patient's words, we are always taking account of the expression of bodies: protest needs to increase the volume of one's voice, focusing on issues that matter – hunger in this case is a sensation of the body, a need for food. It is within the therapeutic session that Anna can show, for the first time in her life, her anger and her hunger. Rather than being narrative, the therapeutic work with her deals with moral agency, the fact that the subject is dignified by her/his own actions. In their chapter Britt and Esther address this by pointing to the complexity assembled in genograms. Genograms tend to be used as snapshots, in their depiction ignoring the relational complexity. In her chapter, Britt considers kinship positions as fluid and multi-stranded layers of events, layers through which the processes of relating fold with history, politics and economics, as well as with the emotions and feelings which are evoked in and through them.

Therapy has inevitably to deal with ethics, it is an ethical operation. The symptom, according to systemic thinking, doesn't take away moral agency from the subject, there is a respect for dignity which prevails over anything else; the dominant psychiatry often takes dignity away through the process of diagnosis and hospitalization.[2]

The English word "assemblage", the translation of the French *agencement*, is used by Deleuze and Guattari (1994) to highlight the agency of connecting together different parts of a "body". Whatever one means with such a word – *agencement* – it is always in connection with action. Assemblage in therapy means also to disassemble the sequences of a narrative, to reassemble them creating *chaosmosis* – *chaos* and *cosmos*, disorder and order that imbricate (Guattari, 1995). Chaosmosis is noise which creates different orders of sequences, the possibility of reversing time, reshaping words, connecting the un-connectable. Such assemblages have to happen all of a sudden within the therapeutic encounter; the therapist needs to be trained in what Bergson (2009) calls *intuition*, which emerges from *duration*. Duration, the extent of time, is the passing of time that is given a synthesis and felt through an intuition (for example, the pendulum signals the time that passes, the concept of duration emerges from an intuition).

When questioned about his way of doing therapy, Cecchin used to answer that, during the session, as time goes by, he waited for an idea to come, listening to family conversation in front of him. As trainees asked to give an example, he usually answered: "I see a couple desperately fighting in front of me, despite both of them are asking for divorce, I start to think on how much they are attached to each other". Far from being the right answer for everybody, this was the unique and unrepeatable style of a great therapist, not something that can be imitated by anyone else. Complexity means creating difference in repetition, it deals with style (Bateson, 1972).

This begs the question: can style be transmitted? Style is not information – in the traditional sense given to such a word by the "theory of information" – it is rather perturbation, in the sense used by Maturana and Varela (1980). To use their language: the orienter orients the orientee within the orientee's cognitive domain. What matters is the "cognitive domain" and the heart of the orientee. What does it mean? In therapy, as well as in training, what matters is what the orientee – the trainee, or the subject who attends therapy – makes of what happens. This works as in the complexity of the constitution of a work of art. In literature, for example, this procedure is called "free indirect discourse" (Pasolini, 1988), in movie-making "subjective image" (Deleuze, 1983). For Bateson this approximates "grace" and integration (Bateson, 1972).

Intuition is not a mysterious gift that someone has and some do not possess, intuition cannot be transmitted from someone to someone else in an abstract way, it is a matter of making experience (*Erlebnis*). As in Heraclitus, you go into the same river, but the water is constantly different. Intuition then acquires good judgment within the relation with the other. One of the main differences between the artist and the therapist is that the artist is permitted not to be understood immediately, the therapist has to deal with what is going on here and now during the session and has a social mandate for change. For any therapist what Bergson (2009) calls "duration" matters, because it is within the process of duration that an intuition comes up, that the therapist makes an attempt to make connections explicit through the hypothesis process. Intuition means creating connections and proposing them to the clients: it means staying in the process; proposing connections not definitive but proposed with a question mark; not believing them as truths; not looking for a first cause; working on the here and now of the process. Time is what passes in the process of the session, there is no need to go to the past in a linear and deterministic absolute way.

To come back to the exergue of this paragraph, clinical work in psychotherapy takes care of symptoms as signs that allow the identification of their trajectory. Symptoms can have adaptive value, they can be phantoms which guarantee the homeostasis of the system and contemporarily a trial to change, in a personal, familiar, communitarian, social sense. The institutions – psychiatric ward, social services etc. – can displace the symptom, creating new trajectories of homeostasis, for example transforming segmental deliria into paranoia, as in Anna's case. The clinical work – as we envisage it – introduces minimal changes, because we do not believe that symptoms are stable issues, but trajectories: where does the symptom take the one who bears it? Or, better, what does the symptom, within the therapeutic relationship, bring us as a present, as a sign? "Us" being the therapist, the patient, the family, the community, the significant others.

We don't believe that high-impact techniques always work for the best; many times, we have seen the contrary, they work *perfectly* for the worse. What is often missing is the attention to the therapeutic relationship: the ecology of therapy since this seems to come from outside, from a pre-defined set of tools.

In our field, the same path has been followed by Gianfranco Cecchin (1987) who described the possible discomfort coming from the position of neutrality and pleas for curiosity. In our view, a tender curiosity is what unites ethic with the aesthetical domain in the field of therapy. Symptoms can be transformed, creating new connections, and the redefinitions proposed enter into the relational aspects of the encounter. There is also the possibility of being contradicted and disputed by those who attend the session; it happens frequently – including the "quarrel" about the patient's symptomatology, which is subtle, often utilizing indirectly other professionals. Usually, the clinician reacts. In this book we claim that disagreements and critiques are very important elements for change; first of all, they change the therapist's prejudices (Cecchin et al., 1992) and his/her positioning, which both are, in our view, the core of therapeutic change. Therapy cannot change if therapists do not change their attitude and their points of view, their emotions as well. It is not – as in the so-called collaborative practices of the social constructionists – that we do not work for change; paradoxically, such a position is a disguised attitude. We are clear about the contract and don't tell lies to our clients. As therapists we work for change in the context, in our client's relationships and in ourselves, anytime we face the singularity of the encounter. In changing ourselves, inevitably we change the therapeutic relationship and symptoms can be transformed, as in the example of Maria Esther (see Chapter 3): the child mentions butterflies, and the family therapist immediately talks about "mom and dad butterfly", the child screams: "No! Butterflies do not have a family!" What is going on here? The "revolutionary" child is challenging the familism of the family therapist. What lines of flight could we face here: butterflies are insects, they are coleopters, they fly, they have colors, they are products of a metamorphosis etc. All these characteristics could be utilized without making a link to a different domain, the one of "families".

It is full of examples where people who attend therapy present their symptoms in connection with some lines of flight that emerge from the relationship between the clinicians and the clients, which can become paths for change. There are many times when the "dull" therapist – as we all are – does not guess what clients mean, we need to admit this. We critique our pretense of infallibility; we need also a critique of the deception of collecting data to demonstrate the perfection of psychotherapy. Neither is reality a mere question of language, nor is language the constitutive material of reality. We think too much power has been given to language and meaning. Nietzsche already had put us on guard against giving too much attention to the linguistic structure, allowing it to determine our comprehension of the world: "the little reason of thought, the great reason of body" (Nietzsche, 1909).

Requests as Always Changing Issues

Therapists in present times do not relate only with so-called patients, they also deal with the problem-determined-system, composed of all the professionals that rotate around a problem, including a teacher, a pediatrician, a pharmacologist, a social worker, a grouchy aunt and ourselves. When a person, a family or a group starts to attend the sessions, they are not a *tabula rasa.* Every conversation we have is embedded in different discursive practices, which are more or less shared or rejected by someone, the therapist included. It could happen that someone comes with this problem: "I am depressed, and the psychiatrist gave me antidepressant medications that did not work, he said that I am drug-resistant and referred me to you"; how to change, not just the request of the "patient" but also all the participants' prejudices? How to transform the relation between a patient and a professional into a therapeutic relationship? How not to undermine the definition given by the psychiatrist, that medications were needed and can't be utilized? The challenge is multiple: first of all, it is the subject who challenges the therapist arriving with two contemporary needs, to change and to remain the same. The observing system is what the professional and/or consultant build together with clients as a context in which to address the problem and the stories that turn around it. Clinicians deal with a multiplicity of events and feelings and can only talk about partial relationships, connections between parties; they need to keep the underlying multiplicities open, always remaining available for new connections. The option to add people in the therapy room remains possible, since it is complexity that explains simplicity and allows for differences and new points of view to emerge. Therapy is not something that happens between two subjects, two or more people, it is an accident that bursts in, an instant that has the power to disarm what is armed and is brought to attention by all the participants. The reference is not only to families – we refuse an exasperated familism – we tend to introduce the economic system and the social one. Even if a volcano is erupting it could have a meaning for the problem-determined system.

Realities are always in becoming. Becoming is a change in the way of relating to the habitual elements of our existence. We are confronted with evolutive and static problem constructions, questions that open up potentialities or that close up options, reifying the statement of the problem itself. We can try to dissolve the problem by redefining it and by not buying it as it was brought to us. It is better if we don't accept the problem as it is stated but if we question the premises that have organized it. The problem is often brought to us as a simple definition in the relationship between history and becoming, the problem/risk is to subordinate becoming to history, instead of keeping reality in parenthesis (Maturana, 1988). Therapy is a particular kind of relationship; it is not parenthood nor friendship. It is a second-order process in which as professionals we don't answer just what comes to our mind or what our heart tells us, we interact and reflect on what we say and do, dealing with what we think is useful for the other. A second-order process means that it is a reflective process in which we interpret our interpretations, we take into consideration the categories we are utilizing and we monitor the cure process: we take care of the cure/care process and of our participation in it.

Therapy is therefore very different from friendship or parent/sister/brother-hood; the affective exchanges, the care and tenderness have the particular shape of being reflexive gestures, not totally spontaneous. They are also temporary gestures, as dissipative structures, designated to continually change and disappear all along, as time goes by, although any one of us professionals will maintain in her/his memory the tender contacts that happened in the past. The encounter is a dissipative structure – a primrose would be joy forever, a rose is a rose but it fades. A work of art is a dissipative structure that evokes stability that goes beyond the author, it transcends him/her (Deleuze and Guattari, 1994); psychotherapy is as well a transient process, but something remains in memory. It is such a tenderness in memory that helps us remember even after 20 years, when the person calling says: "I am … do you remember me?" "Let me think, are you the person who I saw 20 years ago? The one who consulted me because your child was diagnosed encopretic?" "Yes, now he is 28, and fine! I'm calling for another reason". Immediately the affective link re-emerges; therapists are dogs, like Argo, who immediately recognizes Ulysses in the beggar's clothes.

One has to claim that therapy, rather than being interaction, should be envisaged as *intra-action*, what happens simultaneously between two or more subjects/actors on the scene (interactions assumes the anterior existence of independent entities, as Barad suggests (2003)). Therapists are not selling services within a free market; clinic in psychology is neither a shop, nor a court. All people in a therapeutic process – professionals included – are entangled within an irreducible liaison in-between love and economic exchange (Bataille, 1976). Our expertise consists in becoming all part of the same becoming, in order to make realities and possibilities emerge, in order to allow the sense of what actions become possible and which actions we should reject. It is a state of interdependence and involvement among two or more subjects/situations, which react in the immediate as if they were part of the same whole. This makes it possible for us to transform our positioning from up/down into one of curiosity (Cecchin, 1987), which makes the subjects who attend therapy experts by experience.

The beginning of therapy cannot be equal (Barbetta, 2018), this idea is a naïve trick. People who attend therapy pay therapists, directly or indirectly, and ask for our expertise. We are experts of the changing process, clients are experts of their lives; the relationship starts unequal even if organized by mutual respect, and while it proceeds it becomes more and more equivalent, until the clients no longer need to reflect with us on their problems.

As therapists, we need to analyze the quest for therapy (Telfener, 2018). We think that the request people make to us is the last move of a game that includes the symptom; the request has been organized by the same premises that brought the symptom. The person that makes the first call is possibly looking for an ally to endorse his/her positioning (Selvini Palazzoli, 1985) or believes that therapy is needed for some in the system and not for all. We need to analyze the request, to find out what the family members have been doing until now concerning the problem they come in with and what are the motivations that brought them to us, which resources will we be able to rely on. We ask for the resources they can put into the game in order to start the evolution; we then need to not accept the problem as it has been stated until now. We need to reframe the problem, since its current definition is constructed by the same premises that have also organized the symptom and leaving the request with no redefinition makes it harder to create a becoming setting (Ugazio, 1989).

The issue coming from the above considerations definitely claims that it is not the therapist who, alone, changes the request of the "patient" in order to shape it to become evolutive. The quest is an always changing process involving also the therapist; if the therapist doesn't change the premises, if s/he accepts the mandate without redefinition, if s/he accepts the point of view of the majority of professionals and the diagnosis without reflection, the therapeutic system gets stuck, and iatrogenesis develops.

What We Consider Change: The Creation/Production of the New

We are not talking about healing, we don't bring back people to the *status quo ante*, we don't restore what was before. The issue is about creation: the generative process – we free processual and multiplicative forces, oriented to the future rather than to the past. We are not proposing a dogmatic realism but rather a construction of alternatives. Our chore is to open the underlying multiplicities and uncover the potentialities that emerge within the relationships; any relationship reconfigures, re-signifies, changes meaning, positionings and relations. Therapy does the same, in a second-order way: it creates different assemblages, new folds, unfolding and folding again and again the relationship of cooperation between heterogeneous elements, which share a territory. If we follow Bergson, there is no past or future, just a non-linear, not spatial time; time is movement, duration and intensity. We question which lines of flight are present or can be built, we look for them, we elicit them, we use them when we imagine them. Flight lines de-territorialize and re-territorialize elsewhere. According to Bateson a *plateau* is a continuing intensive stabilization. Our way of living in modern Western societies reinforces the idea that we have a tendency to create circuits like those of symmetrical climbing with consequent climax and new beginnings; that there are micro-political forces that lead to programmed lives that repeat themselves over and over. This means that the modalities of intervention on behaviors that we consider socially inappropriate are the imposition of limits. There is another way of thinking: regulations are possible and can maintain the relationship at an acceptable, meta-stable intensity, without climax: new/different ways of interacting, different ways of feeling and behaving. Thinking one or the other way has important consequences for clinical practice.

Conclusions

Psychotherapy is an act of creation, a work of art, or if you prefer, and more modestly, a kind of artisanship based on ethic and aesthetic. It constitutes difference in repetition. It is a praxis that accepts alterity and equivocation as conditions of possibility.

Taking the others seriously means accepting their ontological truths, their reality, their difference; equivocation does not impede relationship, it is rather its condition of possibility, its ontology. Therapy is about partialities that never become a whole: the singular in multiplicity; it is experiencing rather than representation. Systemic clinicians enable the creation of new relationships and territories. In the new world we are facing, it is necessary to clear the ground of pairs such as subject/object; animate/inanimate; human/animal, to wander in uncharted territories of errancy. We need a clinic of the small, tender gesture, that fleeting gesture that might go unnoticed. A tiny gesture, a happening that catches our attention and provokes us, veering from the functional to the expressive. An involuntary purposeless gesture. The difference that makes a difference in repetition. A distinctive feature of art, of life as creation and an act of political resistance.

Notes

1 Umberta is the supervisor, the therapist is a student in her fourth year of training.
2 For the DSM pedophilia and sadism are on the same level as masochism and fetishism; the first two remove moral agency and are not symptoms, they are crimes: there can be no consensus in any case.

References

Barad, K. (2003). Humanist performativity: Toward an understanding of how matter comes to matter. *Signs: Journal of Women in Culture and Society*, 28(3), 801–831.

Barbetta, P. (2018). The unequal exchange: from Ulysses to Shylock. *Human Arenas*. https://doi.org/10.1007/S42087-018-0037-3

Bataille, G. (1976). *La limite de l'utile: ecrits posthumes 1922–1940*, Vol. 7. Milan: Adelphi.

Bateson, G. (1972). *Steps to An Ecology of Mind: Collected Essays in Anthropology, Psychiatry, Evolution, and Epistemology*. Chicago, IL: The University of Chicago Press.

Bergson, H. (2009). *Opere 1889–1896: materia e memoria*. Bari: Laterza.

Blake, W. (1997). *Jerusalem: The Emanation of the Giant Albion. The Illuminated Books of William Blake*, Vol. 1. Princeton, NJ: Princeton University Press (First published 1804).

Cecchin, G. (1987). Hypothesizing, circularity and neutrality revisited: An invitation to curiosity. *Family Process*, 26, 405–413.

Cecchin, G., Lane, G. and Ray, W. (1992). *Irreverence: A Strategy for Therapists' Survival*. London: Karnac.

Deleuze, G. (1983. *Cinema 1: The Movement-Image*. Minneapolis, MN: University of Minnesota Press.

Deleuze, G. and Guattari, F. (1994). *What is Philosophy?* New York: Columbia University Press.

Facchinelli, E. (1983). *Claustrophilia*. Milan: Adelphi.

Foucault, M. (2008). *Psychiatric Power, Lectures at the Collège de France*. London: Picador.

Guattari, F. (1995). *Chaosmosis, an Ethicoaesthetic Paradigm*. Indianapolis, IN: Indiana University Press (First published 1992).

Maturana, H. (1988). Reality: The search for objectivity or the quest for a compelling argument. *Irish Journal of Psychology*, 9(1), 25–82.

Maturana, H. and Varela, F. (1980). *Autopoiesis and Cognition*. Berlin: Springer.

Nietzsche, F. (1909). *Thus Spoke Zarathustra*. Trans. by T. Comman. Edinburgh and London.

Pasolini, P.P. (1988). *Heretical Empiricism*. Indianapolis, IN: Indiana University Press.

Selvini Palazzoli, M. (1985). The problem of the sibling as the referring person. *Journal of Marital and Family Therapy*, 11(1), 21–34.

Telfener, U. (2018). The analysis of the request as the main door to interventions. *Context*, 162, 28–30.

Ugazio, V. (1989). L'indicazione terapeutica: una prospettiva sistemico-costruttivista. *Terapia Familiare*, 31, 27–40.

von Foerster, H. (1984). *Observing Systems*. Seaside, CA: Intersystems.

Chapter 8

Babel, Bebel and Other Dangerous Glossolalia

Pietro Barbetta, Maria Esther Cavagnis,
Inga-Britt Krause and Umberta Telfener

This book is coming to an end. We have been working as a collective and we wonder what will happen to our collective in the future. What follows in this chapter are thoughts and preoccupations each of us have and have had and which we think are in the mix. We have been speaking about therapy as a co-evolutionary process where transparency, irreverence, curiosity and openness are fundamental, where responsibility becomes the way to act ethically. Psychotherapy as philosophy, art, science is considered by us as a discipline which creates and invents. It creates and invents concepts, connections, imagos, actions, potentialities that do not exist already made in a sort of a sky or in a cupboard. In order for them to emerge there must be the necessity to make new links arise, look for consonances, make hypotheses; to set a common goal, a setting, a contract and many other operations. Therapy is an act of creation, in the middle between the axe and the tree of Bateson, between the orchid and the bee of Deleuze, a poetry contest where people have to invent to answer our questions, taking a distance from their usual script, as von Foerster used to say (1984). One "arrives in the middle of something" – as Deleuze states (1983) – "and only in the middle one creates, giving new directions, bifurcations to pre-existing lines". Therapy becomes an interactive, dialogical, performative, second-order, recursive process (contemporarily science and art), in which we touch each other, explore present, past and future within a significant relationship, without goal-directed planning.

Endgame (Maria Esther)

The questions that we used to play by in clinical practice no longer make sense. Questions related to the participants (Who's talking? How many are they? Who's the therapist? Who's the patient? What marks the beginning and the end of that interaction? How many voices are there? How many languages are spoken?); the content (What are they talking about? Their dreams? Their experiences? The rash, the perspiration: are they experiences in themselves or a response to experience?); the interpretation (What is it all about? Was it a

DOI: 10.4324/9780429437410-8

traumatic experience? What is a reactive depression? An unresolved loss? Survivor's guilt?) have no more meaning. We asked ourselves, who's talking? What is he/she saying? What does it mean?

The question today is: How does it work? What is the machination?

We do not choose to think or create. We think and move because we are forced to do so. Forced by what or whom? What is it that forces us away from immobility out of trapped desire? Is it life that drives us to lines of flight in order to escape, to resist? In the face of the infinite singular possibilities of expression of the living, the idea of wholeness in systemic theory now seems to have become a further constraint: a concept bound to the idea of structure, in which relationships are mutually dependent and interior to the whole. Thus development becomes the only possible outcome. Everything is connected, we used to say. Everything that exists is in a relationship to everything else. Today we would say everything is not necessarily connected to everything else. Nor are there totalities that are connected one to the other. Relationships are partial and multiple. Every one part of something may be part of another thing, in a rhizomatic connection.

Lewis Carroll's Alice experiences de-familiarization of the familiar as she leaps out of a room she has lost interest in, through the looking glass, into a world of difference and possibilities: an apt metaphor for our own experience on first reading Deleuze and Guattari. We found ourselves in chaos and, later on – revisiting Bateson, inevitably, as it were a sort of ritornello – in uncharted existential territory yet with the ethical/aesthetic and political potency of their thinking. It was in this search that the meeting took place and we built this Cyborgroup: that ambiguous, heterogeneous creature, half real, half fictional. We come from different countries, cultures, different worlds. We speak different languages. And yet we are connected to each other by multiple affinities as well as the challenge to find common ground, despite the difference, actually upholding that difference. The pre-text was the writing of this book for publication. What actually happened was at once an intense experience of connection and disconnection, communication and in-communication.

Complexity (Pietro)

I propose a way of considering complexity. This is something that, all throughout the meetings of myself with the other three authors, became more and more important. I found myself to be very much in love with the lemma "theory of complexity": my heart beats for Morin (2008), Maturana (2020), Ceruti and Bocchi (1997) and other masters of such a theory. At the same time my heart beats also for Boscolo, Cecchin, Hoffman and Penn (1987) and the proposal not to fall in love with your own ideas. I would like to change the lemma from "theory of complexity" to "aesthetic of complexity". What do I mean now by complexity? The answer is probably the same as Augustin's (2008) when asked about "time": "If they do not ask me, I know it, if they ask me, I am baffled". If one could answer the question "what is complexity" one would reduce it to single items, bits of knowledge, going back to simplification. There is no handbook for complexity. Nonetheless, one can try to imagine some of the issues that deal with complexity, such as for example *emergence* (De Landa, 2016).

One of the senses of *emergence* is that inside knowledge there are discontinuities, or gaps. For example, it is impossible to reduce our thoughts and even our feelings to the flux of neurotransmitters; drugs can change – and not always – something in the physiology of the nervous system, but drugs do not change our thoughts, sometimes not even our feelings. Similarly, therapy can help people to recover new positive feelings and thoughts about life, but not influence people to vote for the Democratic Party. Any field of knowledge has to do with "ontology", which means that there are conditions for our existence. Consider Gorgias's (1971) speech in the *Encomium of Helena*, when he uses the word *pharmakon* to talk about discourse. When Gorgias presents the discourse in terms of *pharmakon* (drug), he does not use a metaphor, he means that discourses have pragmatic effects on people, that people can change in different ways: taking a drug or listening to a discourse. Nonetheless they change in different ways, and they can change for the better or for the worse.

Emergence for me has to do with what emerges out of many possibilities that we don't know beforehand, and has to do with the context and the particular people playing together.

Complexity deals also with *interdisciplinarity*: any item of our knowledge is interconnected with the others: biology with psychology, psychology with politics, art and so forth, despite the tidy organization of disciplines, for example in the academic field.

Another aspect of complexity is *heterogenesis between origin and function* (Darwin, 2020; Foucault, 2001; Nietzsche, 2009). *Genealogy* is the way we search for the origins of something, which has, here and now, a function. Theory has to take into account *things that work*, or *do not*, it has nothing to do with *their origins*. So, what matters in theory – differently from archeology – is not the finding of the origins. This is an important aspect that brings me to talk about *aesthetic*: a theory must be utilizable, aesthetic deals with contemplation, ecstasy.

The *unconscious as a working machine* is another aspect of complexity; it deals with two English words: "function", again, and "work". Work and function are strictly connected: one works to produce a product; if the work is operative or reliable, a good or a service are produced, something useful. In contrast, the work of the unconscious is not what its work produces; it is not a question of working out. The unconscious produces no products, it is a useless working machine, or, better, it has the privilege of being superfluous (Barbetta, 2018).

Another quality of complexity is *singularity*. It is what Descartes calls "admiration" (Irigaray, 1984) and the Greek philosophers call "marvel" or *taumàzein*: "This feeling of wonder shows that you are a philosopher, since wonder is the only beginning of philosophy" (Plato, 2006, *Theaetus.*, 155 d). However, the difference between traditional philosophy and the aesthetic of complexity consists in the fact that philsophy generalizes while aesthetics, as in poetry, approaches singularity in the minute particulars; as in William Blake's plea for good: "General good is the plea for the scoundrels, hypocrite and flatterer" (Blake, *Jerusalem the Emanation of the Giant Albion*, Chapter 3, Plate 55).

Are there other qualities that characterize complexity? Probably infinite others, as hard scientists, social scientists, epistemologists and other scientists have described much better than me; but, for the moment, I am content with the ones mentioned above. I think that they define what it is needed in term of practice: art, praxis, *techne*, as we all wrote in the introduction of this book.

Psychotherapists are practitioners (such a horrible term!), nonetheless their practice deals with the interweaving and interconnection between art and science. Have male therapists the capability to realize their own positioning as "bodies that matter" within a session of a heterosexual couple? What can a woman therapist do in order not to be intimidated by the arrogance of a male patient? How to understand what it means for a Youruba woman to be under a voodoo spell? Or for a practicing Jew, in a Christian country, to be forced to work on Shabbat? Which kind of research does therapy need, in these cases? Using a simple relativist approach one can even think that for any "category" of "client", or "patient", one needs a "category" of therapist: woman with women, male with males, black therapist for black people, Jew with Jewish people, and so on. This would be a terrible reduction of complexity. Nonetheless, if complexity is an aesthetic issue, it cannot be reduced by definition, the politics of complexity can just deal with "minute particulars".

As far as I understand, some professionals argue that there are two different meanings of the word "relativism": one has to do with relativism in philosophy and is a way of saying that we don't believe in one real reality; the other meaning has to do with universalism versus relativism and is utilized by some therapists to talk about a narrow idea that any culture needs a therapist of the same culture. Let's not forget that a mistake of clinicians is to be too universalist and think that *schizophrenia* is the same in the whole world or that the way of curing a young boy in Senegal should be judged by European psychiatrists and follow a Western way of cure.

I agree just in part with my colleague's position I am reporting here (I hope to be faithful to their thoughts). In mental health, we are entangled into the Scilla of radical relativism (represented by hyper-culturalism therapists) and radical universalism (represented by radical biologists in the field of psychiatry). The "fifth province" – to quote Imelda McCarthy and Gail Simon (2016) – is perspectivism.

Incidentally, "perspectivism" is a word used, with the same Deleuzian purpose, by Eduardo Viveiros de Castro in anthropology. This joins my work and practice with Britt's. Part of my work has been, and still is, among asylum seekers, as is Britt's clinical anthropological practice at the Tavistock in London. It is a pity that few psychologists and family therapists of present days know so little or nothing of the anthropological terminology and meanings. I think that we are also fighting a "battle" in our field in order to teach clinical anthropology to our students – I think it is an essential antidote to disentangle therapists from familism (Deleuze and Guattari, 1983). As in Bateson's teaching: meanings come from differences that make a difference, not from homogeneity.

The Ontological Turn (Britt)

Shall we go back to the beginning? – We cannot, because there is no beginning – or rather there are many beginnings! Sharing is at the end of the process rather than at the beginning. Our starting point is thus not universals, because universals "explain nothing and must themselves be explained" (Deleuze and Guattari, 1991, p. 7). Nor can the starting point be concepts because "you will know nothing through concepts unless you have first created them" (Deleuze and Guattari, 1991, p. 7). Ingold says: "To have in common is not to look inside ourselves, to regress to a set of baseline attributes with which we are similarly endowed from the start, but to reach out to others who are... different from us" (Ingold, 2017, pp. 14–15).

So in this last chapter let us go to something which we may consider our prologue. Bateson was ahead of his time, in anticipating the Ontological Turn (Holbraad and Pedersen, 2017), but since the discovery was late in the days of the Naven work, and since no one really has read *Naven* anyway, perhaps it is understandable that this was forgotten about and that systemic psychotherapists have had difficulty in keeping in mind "perspective" as well as the full implications of cultural differences, or even just of difference itself, despite this being one of our central preoccupations. These difficulties have had implications for the way thinking and practicing with other ideas such as "relationship", "genogram" and "system" have developed in our discipline.

The *Ontologial Turn* is an approach in social anthropology which takes difference seriously. It suggests that what differs is not just epistemologies, i.e. how we access what there is or how we understand what there is, but also that "reality" itself can be different to different people and in different situations. In this way there is not just one, colonial, objective ontology, but many ontologies. There are several other great authors, von Foerster, Maturana and in a different way Foucault, who share this premise even if they each take this in slightly different directions. This must also sound OK to some of you! At least those of you who are social constructionists must be wanting to shout "Hurray!" But wait a minute – how does this work? There are, as one would expect, differences within the Ontological Turn itself and my invitation is to you, audience (and readers), to engage with what you might want the

Ontological Turn to look like in systemic psychotherapy, since ours is a discipline in which practice is theoretical practice as well as practice theory.

Above we alluded to "sharing" or "communicating". Our name for this is "relationship". What is this? How do we understand the concept of "relationship"? Bateson's idea of schismogenesis was groundbreaking and suggested that a relationship is an exchange in which there is something of each party in the other without them becoming one. This is so in two senses. First, because there is an exchange, could be of physical things, stuff, emotions, thoughts etc., and second, because as a result of social conventions – of occupying the same space, being in the room together – the two parties are already related and they are, as it were, keeping or thickening this relation with more and new layers and rounds of exchange. Strathern said that "persons have relations integral to them" (Strathern, 2004, p. 101). Parties to a relationship therefore have "two views of the same thing", and the exchange and reciprocity is in fact an exchange of perspectives (Wagner, 1981). In other words, "the way is not the same in both directions" (Viveiros de Castro, 2017). Since "perspective" implies multiplicity, with persons we have multiplicities, which are different from essences (Deleuze, 1994). What is emerging is a different view of "person" and "relationship" than that which seems to operate in most depictions of genograms and families in our discipline. In Roy Wagner's words, persons are fractal, by which he means that: "A fractal person is never a unit standing in a relation to an aggregate, or an aggregate standing in relation to a unit, but always an entity with relationships integrally implied" (Wagner, 1981, p. 163). Strathern talks about persons and relations being "partial connections" (Strathern, 2004). There exists then in any relationship two poles, the actual (what Deleuze calls the "extensive") pole, which refers to the relationship as described in cultural, social, political and linguistic terms, and the virtual (Deleuze calls this the "intensive") pole, which contains within it the possibility for going forward. In this sense the virtual is greater than the real, so that actualizing the virtual involves selecting from the real and limiting it.

This account is a simplification, but we hope you the reader get the gist. Could we get any further away from the concept of the single autonomous individual or person of Western psychology which dominates thinking in systemic psychotherapy today? What then might be the implications of the view I have put forward?

One implication of the fractal person, of the multiplicities in the potential for perspectives in relationships, is that we must bear in mind that a person occupies simultaneously many positions in line with what is available on the extensive plane. So a mother is also a sister, a daughter, a grandmother and a wife / female partner. A father is also a brother, a son, a husband / male partner. A child is a son or a daughter, a brother/sister, a father/mother, uncle/ aunt, a grandfather/grandmother and so on. At any given time no one is all these at once, "but each at terminal points of the distance over which he or she glides" (Viveiros de Castro, 2017). This derives from inspiration from Lévi-Strauss and interpretations by Deleuze and Viveiros de Castro, and was originally cast in terms of particular non-Western kinship systems. However we may make use of this in terms of understanding the positions from which a client speaks and is not so foreign for us if we bear in mind our traditions of teaching life cycles and the development of domestic groups: a mother may speak as a daughter or as a sister – any kinship position takes on a multiplicity of available other partial connections without these being considered "biological givens". A mother does not need to be a biological mother in order to take up a position of a "mother". Rather positions are made available on the extensive plane in the dynamic between the real and the virtual. With this view comes a breakdown of the bounded system, which the family is frequently assumed to be. Rather as Deleuze and Guattari suggest, "every conceptual distinction begins with the establishment of an extensive-actual pole and an intensive-virtual one. The relationship is one of "reciprocal presupposition in which one pole is always described as a version or transformation of the other" (Viveiros de Castro, 1991, p. 119). But importantly this is an asymmetrical reciprocity: the way is not the same in both directions! There are two movements, one at the extensive/actual pole where there is a decline of differences of potential, and one at the intensive/virtual pole, which is the creator of difference. This latter movement is what Deleuze calls "becoming". This is process, not system.

Another implication is a questioning of bringing everything back to language, of language as a force in itself. In *Difference and Repetition*, Deleuze (1994) poses the question of "what does it means to think" in a way which is very different from the way this was posed by Descartes. Rather than considering "thinking" as defining our existence, the suggestion is that it is "the encounter", which because it is sensed in our bodies and with our emotions, is the pre-condition for thought and thinking. The therapeutic encounter is of course one example of this, and once in it we the therapist have a relationship with our clients. So we therapists too are fractal persons, with partial connections and multiple perspectives in which it is never the same in both directions. Words, meaning, texts and representations generally, while inescapable and important therapeutic tools, cannot capture these multiplicities which Deleuze considers "the irreducible inequality of difference and that forms the condition of the world" (Deleuze, 1994, p. 222) (this is the image of the rhizome).

Whatever the critics (Graeber, 2015), the Ontological Turn takes "difference" seriously and for this reason alone merits the attention of systemic psychotherapists. Holbraad and Pedersen say "To 'take the ontological turn' seriously... means that the concepts by which a given ethnographic encounter is analysed must be in ontological continuity with this encounter" (Holbraad and Pedersen, 2017, p. 286). This is a very clear (and systemic) statement about the centrality of process when working with relationships.

Reflecting on a Case (Umberta)

Renato is a 22-year-old young man who arrives to my office after a call from his father in September 2019; they are sent to me from a colleague of the mother. His father is a physicist, the mother a psychiatrist, he has a brother of 19 years old still in school. I invite the whole family but the father asks me to see R. alone, since they already tried to go as a family and "it did not work". I comply, thinking I will be able to invite everybody in the near future, and I greet R. who is a very good looking guy. Dark hair, green eyes, thin, he tells me he has just missed the occasion of his life, since he was on a Truman Show and had the possibility to gain a lot of money, millions of euros. He has been fired because he had not understood the contract and called the organizers names by phone and internet. He was famous and people in the street were recognizing him and speaking about him, because they had seen him on the show.

I understand during the first session that I don't want to follow the path of the Truman Show: he believes in this narrative and doesn't want to let it go. I therefore tell him I need to know him better and ask permission to abandon for a moment "his obsession": without disqualifying him, I need to know him better. After having drawn a genogram with him, I decide to reason on the money issue that must be a family theme.

> "Not to have money, the risk of losing money, is it an issue in your family, Renato?"
> "Absolutely. Father is always afraid that there's no money in the family, he is exaggerating. It has been happening since mother and father has separated two years ago".
> "You worry about money too?"
> "No, I don't think so. I lost this millionaire contract and feel stupid and desperate. I am full of regrets".

I then become interested in his daily life. What does he do, apart from living with regrets? Not much, he works in a supermarket and tries to study physics. He has never kissed a girl, has never dated, lives half the time with father in a tiny town 40 miles from Rome and the other half with mother who just moved to Rome, where he goes to university. I like R. but feel fidgety about where to go with him. He would like to talk only about the Truman Show, since he does not talk about it at home, nor with the few people he meets. I feel it is useless, a loss of time, a way of "watering" his symptom and making it flourish.

In a cybernetic-systemic epistemology, the therapist doesn't know better and more than the client: her theories, her hypotheses, her comments are not true or false, they are exactly as plausible as the ones of the client. What differentiates the two positions is that the professional's hypotheses are on a different logical order: not at the content level of what one thinks, they are interwoven in the processes which builds how we think, perceive and decide. Not at the first-order level of "understanding", but rather at the second-order level of "understanding our understanding" and "knowing about knowing" (Bianciardi and Telfener, 2014). My inevitably prejudiced reflections state that a highly obsessed young man needs to get distracted from his obsession – that I feel very boring and repetitive – and contemporarily that we need to find an area to work on that can be of success: girls, study, new friends in Rome could be themes to explore. My thoughts and feelings bring me to feel frustrated and hesitant, I thus decide that the relationship with him should come before anything else. I wish for a light and smiley rapport in which we simultaneously can joke and be serious.

The therapist brings with herself the bits and pieces of her own existence and acts purposefully, not to bring the system from A to B, but to create a morphogenetic field (Sheldrake, 2011) in which to share an unconscious and a common intent that is evolutionary. This field is made of the two of us, of his family, even if I have not yet met them, and of all the people that interact around Renato, their intentions, presuppositions, ideas, feelings and desires. We belong to a common unconscious that was just created. I therefore try to find out who else is in the picture and which diagnoses were named. Renato's mother is a psychiatrist, and he has gone to see a psychiatrist – sent by her – but now he is not taking the medication they gave him nor does he seem worried about the words "psychosis" and "delirium" that were mentioned by the ward where he stayed for three days after having a violent tantrum and destroying his room.

Therapy works on the presence, without proposing a beginning or an end. The process allows the clinician to describe what she was able to see. Experimenting instead of affirming, problematizing, cartographing, designing temporary maps, making connections emerge. I feel he is caught between two loyalties, between father and mother, and explore this hypothesis:

"Was the separation among your parents harsh? Did they fight much?"
"No, their separation came out of the blue. We did not know they were intending to separate. They told us when everything was already decided. The next day they started to live apart".
"Did you feel you needed to take sides?"
"No. Mother has a work she loves and is excited to start living in Rome; father keeps his job going and is very secluded. He studies a lot".
"Two different styles of life. Did you ever feel you needed to choose which one yours would be?"
"No. I have my own life".
"What kind of life?"
"I could have been rich, if I respected the unspoken contract".

Exploring further I find out that Renato in his town – his father's town – goes to a bar near home and smokes dope and drinks heavily with two companions: the fruit stand worker and the bar attender ("Do I have the power in the first session to speak about the use of dope?" I think to myself; "No" I answer). Rome is the town of discipline, he has no friends from the university, apart from a few study companions that he meets only during class hours ("This kid is left too much on his own" I think to myself); he has also lost all his school friends since he changed his style of life.

My way seems blocked by his many "NOs". Actually I continue feeling that Renato has no ground, no roots, as if this family was just the agglomeration of four people sharing a place that we should not yet call home. A hypothesis needs to make un-thought questions, connections, new problems emerge. I wish to multiply interactions and emotions, I need to free thought and emotions, I must not be afraid. I therefore start asking for family tales, anecdotes that involve also the grandmothers and one aunt. Renato seems very vague, he remembers very little, he certainly is not a storyteller. Could he come next session with his family in order to explore the family humus, the atmosphere in which he has grown up? He doesn't seem happy about my proposal, but accepts to ask both parents to come in; he would like to leave brother at home, in order not to share his "secret" with him. Happy that his reality of the Truman Show has become "a secret" – although I feel everybody knows what is happening – I decide that he deserves a moment with parents on his own and comply with his request. "Is it a collusion?" I ask myself, and answer that it is not if I act not out of fear but do it in a strategizing modality, in order to create a relationship with Renato.

I am not suggesting looking for novelty in itself, but rather to hypothesize where to look and what to look for; I intend to send probe balloons and consider what comes back. The feedback I receive becomes very important. I know that new is unattended and often irreverent, new is always unforeseen, it is made of little details that pass by unnoticed thoughts and feelings that invade and take the place of anxiety and rumination.

The therapist actively utilizes herself and her abilities to connect. Contrarily to others around him, I did not look worried when he mentioned hashish and am not judgmental about his symptom. I feel Renato likes me and stays with me in the here and now. I am proposing a multiple positioning, not so much of different kinds of *capta*, but rather a manifold point of view which combines: 1) the consideration of the context in which we are acting; 2) the observation of the asymmetrical but equal relationship established between the client and the professional and their reference systems; 3) a study of the client and his significant relationships; 4) a reflection on the generativity of the process, on the poetics that emerges from what has been proposed, said and done. The context (1) is a private office with little interference from the outside and no other professionals for the moment involved in the case, even the one who sent it to me doesn't seem involved. Our relationship (2) is one of trust even if I feel that what I say has no impact on Renato and we don't share any hypothesis on the meaning and the reason of his distress. Renato invites at a session his parents (3) and they seem in a big conflict, with mother strong and outspoken and father weak and silent. He regrets the separation from his wife and walks around home talking to himself and complaining about a loss of money, that according to the other two is only due to stressful anxiety. Is Renato trying to protect father keeping mother involved, is he acting as "the glue" between the two? Is he showing father that there are "real" reasons and serious ones for losing money? Has he a secret alliance with father and from father has inherited the shyness and the social difficulties? Is he just smoking too much dope as the parents claim? Is he testing the context to see who he can trust, or – in the opposite direction – is he trying to have a good reason to seclude himself at home without going out into the vast world? Is he afraid of disappointing mother, as father has? The plausible possibilities are really many, none of which resonate with Renato, who remains within his obsession. Many hypotheses seem acceptable to me, making me incapable of taking a position: in a rigid system it is useful to have one core meaning and bring it forward as a constant around which the whole system must rotate and therefore modify. This seems a semi-rigid system and I allow myself to have more than one hypothesis. The process needs time to become generative (4). It becomes interesting when Renato starts going out with girls: he goes twice to a disco in Rome and is picked up both times by young girls that bring him home for a one night stand. He is thrilled of his new sexual experiences, even if he needs to drink in order to enter the disco; he takes some exams, gets decent grades and starts going out more. The Truman Show slides to the background. We continue talking about richness and poorness: in feelings, in security of self, in experience, in culture and curiosity.

To perturb in therapy means to create events, make things happen, utilize words, movement and space. As therapists we make an act of resistance. We need to be irreverent, produce something not expected, not recognized: the capacity to think outside of the box. For approximately seven months we go on seeing each other every 15 days, the Truman Show remains in the background and we seem not to need to talk about it. Renato never stated clearly that it was an obsession or a delirium, until the end of July 2020 when he calls me to say that he feels he is very confused: "My head smokes" – he tells me – "I am afraid to screw everything up. An electrical short circuit has occurred. I need help". He arrives to my office and tells me his obsessive thoughts are back, the Truman Show as well, but this time he believes it is a sign of anxiety and not "reality". We look for the triggering event and we both agree that it could be a girl he was courting through Whatsapp during lockdown who has disappeared.

We start again to meet weekly. But this is another story.

Coming to the End (Maria Esther)

Psychotherapy is a creative act based on an aesthetic that constitutes an affirmation of difference. It can no longer be viewed as a problem arising from language, a representation or a social construct. It is rather a new praxis that:

- Accepts alterity and equivocation as conditions of possibility.

  "Taking the other seriously" means accepting their ontological truths, their reality, their difference. Equivocation does not impede relationship, it is rather its founding and driving principle: difference as perspective. A condition of possibility at the boundary of the therapeutic effort.

- It rejects the empire of the one and only.

  It's about partialities that never become a whole. The singular in multiplicity. A collective could be thought of as a continuous variation among its heterogeneous elements, the mutual affectation of singular forces. The rule is not to ever allow anyone to speak in the name of everyone.

- It is post-structural: no hierarchy, no form, nor hierarchy of form.
- It is vitalist political action: it works with forces rather than forms; with desire and the capture of desire. Change comes into being as life rids itself of its shackles.
- It is experiencing rather than representation.It is only through our encounters that we discover that which connects with our body to become an organizing relationship, that which suits us, the strength to live, to act, to make us joyful.

- A cartographic clinical practice: its trajectory and effects.

  Rather than the representation of the "known" world, it enables the creation of new relationships and territories, new "machines". In clinical practice we have been compelled to follow the given trajectories. It is necessary to clear the ground of such pairs as subject/object; animate/inanimate; human/animal; conscious/unconscious to wander in uncharted territories of errancy.

- A clinic of the small gesture.

  Paying attention to gesture, that fleeting gesture that might go unnoticed. A tiny gesture, a happening that catches our attention and provokes us, veering from the functional to the expressive. An involuntary purposeless gesture. The difference that makes a difference in repetition. A distinctive feature of art, of life as creation and an act of political resistance.

The Pink Floyd Album *The Dark Side of the Moon* (1973) shows a ray of light that crosses a prism and separates into its fundamental frequencies, becoming something else. It becomes a series of colors that were present but hidden. A plane of immanence. Therapists as well give light to unheard *capta* and we distance ourselves from the blueprint with which the client has come to us.

References

Augustin. (2008). *The Confessions.* Oxford: Oxford University Press.

Barbetta, P. (2018). The unequal exchange: From Ulysses to Shylock. *Human Arenas.* https://doi.org/10.1007/s42087-018-0037-3

Bianciardi, M. and Telfener, U. (2014). *Ricorsività in psicoterapia, riflessioni sulla pratica clinica.* Turin: Bollati Boringhieri.

Boscolo, L., Cechin, G.F., Hoffamn, L. and Penn, P. (1987). *Milan Systemic Family Therapy.* New York: Basic Books.

Ceruti, M. and Bocchi, G. (1997). *La sfida della complessità,* Milan: Feltrinelli.

Darwin, C. (2021). *On the Origin of Species Illustrated.* London: The Folio Society.

De Landa, M. (2016). *Assemblage Theory.* Edinburgh: Edinburgh University Press.

Deleuze, G. (1983). Qu'est-ce que l'acte de creation? https://zintv.org/outil/quest-ce-que-lacte-de-creation-par-gilles-deleuze-1987/

Deleuze, G. (1994). *Difference and Repetition.* London: Bloomsbury.

Deleuze, G. and Guattari, F. (1983). *Anti-Oedipus: Capitalism and Schizophrenia.* Minneapolis, MN: University of Minnesota Press.

Deleuze, G. and Guattari, F. (1991). *What is Philosophy?* New York: Columbia University Press.

Foucault, M. (2001). *The Order of Things.* London: Routledge.

Gorgias (1971). *Works.* London: Penguin.

Graeber, D. (2015). Radical alterity is just another way of saying "reality": A reply to Eduardo Viveiros de Castro. *HAU: Journal of Ethnographic Theory,* 5(2), 1–41.

Holbraad, M. and Pedersen, M.A. (2017). *The Ontological Turn: An Anthropological Exposition.* Cambridge: Cambridge University Press.

Ingold, T. (2017). On human correspondence. *Journal of the Royal Anthropological Institute,* 23(1), 9–27.

Irigaray, L. (1984). *Éthique de la différence sexuelle.* Paris: Minuit.

McCarthy, I. and Simon, G. (2016) *Systemic Therapy as Transformative Practice.* Everything is Connected Press.

Maturana, H. (2020). *El sentido de lo humano.* Santiago de Chile: Paidos Chile.

Morin, E. (2008). *Comprendre la complexité.* Paris: L'Harmattan.

Nietzsche, F. (2009). *On the Genealogy of Morals.* London: Oxford University Press.

Plato. (2006). *Dialogues.* New York: Bantam.

Sheldrake, R. (2011). *The Presence of the Past: Morphic Resonance and the Habits of Nature.* London: Icon Books.

Strathern, M. (2004). *Partial Connections,* updated edn. Oxford: Altamira Press.

Viveiros de Castro, E. (1991). *The Relative Native: Essays on Indigenous Conceptual Worlds.* Chicago, IL: HAU.

Viverios de Castro, E. (2017). *Cannibal Metaphysics.* London: University of Minnesota Press.

von Foerster, H. (1984). *Observing Systems.* Seaside, CA: Intersystems.

Wagner, R. (1981). *The Invention of Culture.* London: The University of Chicago Press.

Postscript

The Event

Pietro Barbetta, Maria Esther Cavagnis,
Inga-Britt Krause and Umberta Telfener

In this postscript we give an account of an event in which the four of us participated. In this event we attempted to demonstrate, communicate and enact the idea that the conditions of representation lie in life, that is to say in a realm outside that which can be put forward in the form of representations or meanings which are generally assumed to capture what life is. We have on occasion, while writing this book, become frustrated at the difficulty of conveying our ideas and thought in language and we think that the event offered a different and perhaps more accessible and evocative view of our writing to our audience. The event took place in the 10th Conference of the European Family Therapy Association in Naples in September 2019 as part of a symposium entitled Ethic and Aesthetic Explorations in Psychotherapy. We performed the event at the opening of the symposium and were then encouraged by the audience to repeat it after the presentations at the end of the symposium. The idea and the performance of the event were loosely inspired by Samuel Beckett's play *Quad* (Beckett, 1992).[1] Beckett has also been extensively commented on by Deleuze (Deleuze, 1997). We had marked out a red square on the floor with sticky tape. Each of us positioned ourselves in a corner of the square. During the performance each of us moved across and along each time one of us spoke. Words and sentences were spoken in turn from a script. We spoke in our different languages: English, Italian (northern), Spanish, Danish, Italian (southern).

The script contained the following words:

BRITT: The time we were in Libya, I came there 2013, so in 2014, there was a war in Libya and during that war that the four of us were working and as we were working, and the bomb fell in our mist. It was closer to the three of them than me, I was a little bit far from them and where the bomb fell. It lifted us all up and then we fell heavily to the ground. It took like an hour for me to gain consciousness, when I opened my eyes, the three other people were dead, I was the only one who survived. When I got up, my phone and everything were broken. So, I went to the friends I had

DOI: 10.4324/9780429437410-9

there. So, after a week, I started seeing rashes on my face like chickenpox and it started turning into sores. I bought of drugs, out of my work I had money to buy lots of drugs, and there (in Libya) you cannot go to the hospital, I bought lots of medicine, so after... when I sleep...

UMBERTA: After that incident, when I sleep, and dream, that scene is the only thing I see, about what happened with me and the three other people I was working with who died. And then when I wake up, am unable to sleep again until daybreak and I will have unbearable headache throughout the day until sunset.

MARIA ESTHER: Si no te molesta, puedes describirme las cosas que ves en tus sueños?

PIETRO: A vedi sti tri amis che ghe lauravi insema, ma dopu fasem un laurà divers de quel normal che fasevum lalàinscì, dopu a moeren ancamò in del sogn. Dopu incuminci a tremà e levi su, dopu rièsi pu a dormì.

MARIA ESTHER: Siempre sueñas lo mismo o a veces tus sueños son diferentes?

UMBERTA: Sogno anche altre cose, anche con gli altri sogni, quando mi sveglio, sento ancora il mal di testa, comunque la cosa che capita più spesso è quella di sognare me stesso con gli altri tre

BRITT: Er der nætter du aldrig drømmer noget, eller drømmer du hver nat?

PIETRO: Some nights I have dreams different from the dreams about me and the three men, but it takes time for me to go back to sleep, for those ones, I can go back to sleep again.

BRITT: Kan du huske en drøm du har drømt for nylig?

UMBERTA: The night before this morning I was with these same three people (the friends who are dead) we were going to some place, we were walking and as we were walking, they ask me to enter into a building, and I said I will not enter, they kept on insisting, and I said no, so one of the center female officials call out my name from behind, and told me not to follow them, and that I should get back, when I turned back, that's when I woke up...

MARIA ESTHER: Fue como si tuvieras miedo

PIETRO: Did you pass through the desert from Ghana to Libya?

BRITT: Yes

UMBERTA: Quanti anni avevi?

MARIA ESTHER: 23. Porque ahora tengo 25. Cuando dejé Libia tenia 23.

We made words circulate from one side to the other, also in reverse. "What happened? How would you comment?" we asked the public who were observing in a participant mode. Many stimuli came through. We spoke then about the uselessness of words, of how meaning comes about, about relatedness and dreams. Here the dream is not at all the typical psychoanalytical dream, it seems more similar to the dream tradition, like Joseph in the Bible or Artemidorus Oneirocritica, or a kind of divination. So the dreams have a different materiality, a different consistency, ontological differences from the classical "interpretation of dreams". Here dreams are the ways to express the sense of the traumatic experience.

We do not pretend to have been able to reproduce Beckett's precise patterns in which colored robes were a central feature creating a pattern and in which the central square remained visible and empty of any movement at all times. Nor did we manage to capture the timelessness of the original play which gives a feeling of no beginning and no ending. In our event we all appeared at the same time in our corners and as we spoke we each moved diagonally across to a colleague who at the same time moved to the right, followed by the person in that corner simultaneously moving to the right, until all the corners were again occupied. The next person to speak initiated the same movement. The pace was not slow but we tried to keep to a steady rhythm and coordination and to speak clearly. We were concerned to demonstrate both synchrony and multiplicity. We hope that we captured a sense of an interconnecting, folding happening with the emergence of interconnections with different starting and ending points in a process rather than a static picture. A kind of "ontological mobility" (May, 2005, p. 122). We were also concerned to de-emphasize both the semiotic and linguistic aspects of language and to convey and capture the circumstances – or rather assemblages – in which we and everyone in the room took part, or to use an expression by Barad were entangled (Barad, 2007). That is to say we wanted to decenter the subject. To our minds, systemic psychotherapy, thanks to the influence of Bateson and the renewal of his ideas both in second-order cybernetics and in contemporary social research, is well positioned to take this project forward. However, with the event and with this book we are also suggesting that while the subject might have been somewhat obscured in systemic psychotherapy, eschewing the subject altogether also obstructs a grasp of the full implications of the primacy of relations over relata (Krause, 2012) and the extent of entanglement of individual events, entities and sets of practices (Barad, 2007). This is why we have been inspired by Deleuze's idea of "the body without organs" (Deleuze, 1990), suggesting that individual human beings may not be the proper ontological units for political, therapeutic, social, cultural or any other enquiry. The event which took place and which we have described here was an attempt to point to a more fluid ontology with more possibilities for change and experimentation.

Note

1 *Quad* is based on a geometrical figure and on permutations of regular movements. First one, then two, then three, then four figures, dancers or mime artists, dressed in colored loose robes (white, yellow, blue and red) appear one after another to scurry along the sides and across the diagonals of a square, shuffling in strict rhythm to a rapid percussion beat. Each figure then departs in the order in which he appeared, leaving another to recommence the sequence... Strikingly all of them avoid the center which is clearly visible in the middle of the square.

References

Barad, K. (2007). *Meeting the Universe Halfway: Quantum Physics and the Entanglement of Matter and Meaning.* Durham, NC: Duke University Press.

Beckett, S. (1992). *Quad et autre pieces pour la télévision.* Paris: Les Éditions de Minuit.

Deleuze, G. (1990). *Logic of Sense.* London: Bloomsbury (First published 1969).

Deleuze, G. (1997). *Essays Critical and Clinical.* Minneapolis, MN: University of Minnesota Press.

Krause, I.-B. (2012). Culture and the reflexive subject in systemic psychotherapy. In I.-B. Krause (ed.), *Culture and Reflexivity in Systemic Psychotherapy: Mutual Perspectives.* London: Karnac Books.

May, T. (2005). *Gilles Deleuze: An Introduction.* Cambridge: University of Cambridge Press.

Index